HIV Treatment - New Developments

Edited by Samuel Okware

Published in London, United Kingdom

HIV Treatment - New Developments
http://dx.doi.org/10.5772/intechopen.107745
Edited by Samuel Okware

Contributors
Alexander Pivnik, Amit Lunkad, Arsen Vukovich, Edwin Kimathi, Gordon Ogweno, Paula Freitas, Sachin Namdeo Kothawade, Samuel Okware, Sara Ribeiro, Vaibhav Wagh, Vishal Pande

First published in London, United Kingdom, 2024 by IntechOpen
IntechOpen is the global imprint of INTECHOPEN LIMITED, registered in England and Wales, registration number: 11086078, 5 Princes Gate Court, London, SW7 2QJ, United Kingdom
Printed in Croatia

British Library Cataloguing-in-Publication Data
A catalogue record for this book is available from the British Library

Additional hard and PDF copies can be obtained from orders@intechopen.com

HIV Treatment - New Developments
Edited by Samuel Okware
p. cm.

This title is part of the Infectious Diseases Book Series, Volume 30
Topic: Viral Infectious Diseases
Series Editor: Alfonso J. Rodriguez-Morales
Topic Editor: Shailendra K. Saxena

Print ISBN 978-1-83769-072-5
Online ISBN 978-1-83769-073-2
eBook (PDF) ISBN 978-1-83769-074-9
ISSN 2631-6188

IntechOpen Book Series
Infectious Diseases
Volume 30

Aims and Scope of the Series

This series will provide a comprehensive overview of recent research trends in various Infectious Diseases (as per the most recent Baltimore classification). Topics will include general overviews of infections, immunopathology, diagnosis, treatment, epidemiology, etiology, and current clinical recommendations for managing infectious diseases. Ongoing issues, recent advances, and future diagnostic approaches and therapeutic strategies will also be discussed. This book series will focus on various aspects and properties of infectious diseases whose deep understanding is essential for safeguarding the human race from losing resources and economies due to pathogens.

Meet the Series Editor

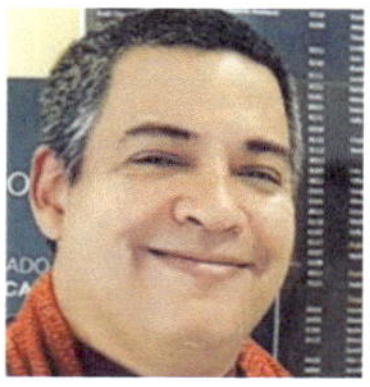

Dr. Rodriguez-Morales is an expert in tropical and emerging diseases, particularly zoonotic and vector-borne diseases (notably arboviral diseases), and more recently COVID-19 and Monkeypox. He is the president of the Publications and Research Committee of the Pan-American Infectious Diseases Association (API), as well as the president of the Colombian Association of Infectious Diseases (ACIN). He is a member of the Committee on Tropical Medicine, Zoonoses, and Travel Medicine of ACIN. Dr. Rodriguez-Morales is a vice-president of the Latin American Society for Travel Medicine (SLAMVI) and a member of the Council of the International Society for Infectious Diseases (ISID). Since 2014, he has been recognized as a senior researcher at the Ministry of Science of Colombia. He is a professor at the Faculty of Medicine of the Fundacion Universitaria Autonoma de las Americas, in Pereira, Risaralda, Colombia, and a professor, Master in Clinical Epidemiology and Biostatistics, at Universidad Científica del Sur, Lima, Peru. He is also a non-resident adjunct faculty member at the Gilbert and Rose-Marie Chagoury School of Medicine, Lebanese American University, Beirut, Lebanon, and an external professor, Master in Research on Tropical Medicine and International Health, at Universitat de Barcelona, Spain. Additionally, an invited professor, Master in Biomedicine, at Universidad Internacional SEK, Quito, Ecuador, and a visiting professor, Master Program of Epidemiology, at Diponegoro University, Indonesia. In 2021 he was awarded the "Raul Isturiz Award" Medal of the API and, the same year, the "Jose Felix Patiño" Asclepius Staff Medal of the Colombian Medical College due to his scientific contributions to the topic of COVID-19 during the pandemic. He is currently the Editor in Chief of the journal Travel Medicine and Infectious Diseases. His Scopus H index is 55 (Google Scholar H index 77) with a total of 725 publications indexed in Scopus.

Meet the Volume Editor

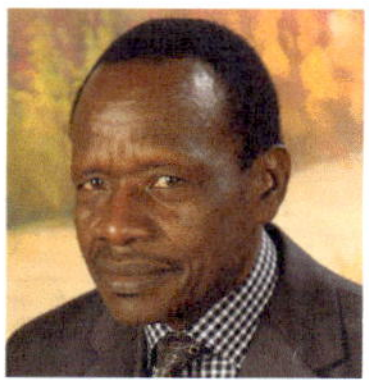

Dr. Samuel Okware is a public health specialist with a Ph.D. in Emerging Infections. He pioneered HIV research and control in Sub-Saharan Africa. His work on HIV/AIDS led to the earliest strategies for HIV prevention, which resulted in significant declines in incidence among key populations. He has spent many years coordinating and leading national public health programs against communicable diseases in Uganda. He served on several technical advisory committees, including the WHO Expert Committee on Research and Development. He is the Director General of the Uganda National Health Research Organization, which coordinates health research in the country. He has received several awards in recognition of his contribution to HIV prevention and control. Dr. Okware has published extensively on HIV and remerging infections.

Contents

Preface

The search for a cure for human immunodeficiency virus (HIV) infection remains a persistent challenge in HIV control and elimination. Increasing advances in technology have led to significant breakthroughs in new treatments, transforming HIV/AIDS from a highly fatal condition to a chronic ailment. It is possible with the current technological momentum to discover a cure for HIV/AIDS. Various classes of highly active antiretroviral drugs are currently available. They include nucleotide reverse transcription inhibitors (NRTIs), non-nucleotide reverse transcriptase inhibitors (NNTRIs), integrase inhibitors, and protease inhibitors. However, these drugs have some challenges and gaps in meeting the global target of elimination of HIV infection by 2030. Most of the concerns for the total eradication of the virus lie in new technologies and therapeutic tools.

The introductory chapter of this book lays the groundwork for consideration of the challenges undermining HIV infection prevention and control. It discusses these gaps and perspectives and urges for a cure as the ultimate tool for attaining the goal of eliminating HIV/AIDS by 2030. The discussion introduces some options for the elimination and suggests gene-based therapies and nanotechnology-based approaches as well as long-acting drugs to enhance access, mitigate resistance, and improve quality of care.

The major challenges of the current treatments for HIV/AIDS are their short life and inability to reach potential reservoirs of infection, especially the central nervous system, lymph nodes, and the lungs, including latently infected cells. In addition, drug toxicity in some patients leads to poor adherence and subsequent drug resistance. There may be an escalation of comorbidities and non-communicable diseases. These limitations have necessitated the exploration of safer and user-friendly drug options for the elimination of the virus to control rebound of viremia once drugs have been stopped.

The second section discusses drug treatments for HIV and their challenges. Against this background, the first chapter in this section discusses the challenges related to the use of antiplatelet therapy in HIV treatment. Routinely, antiplatelet agents are recommended for primary prevention and treatment of individuals at risk of ischemic stroke and heart attack. However, current treatment guidelines and recommendations were developed using data from non-HIV populations. The second chapter reveals the emerging clinical resistance to antiplatelet therapy in the primary prevention and treatment of cardiovascular events in people living with HIV. The systematic review of evidence further reveals that people living with HIV and non-HIV individuals respond differently to antiplatelet remedies. The chapter reviews the effects of individual antiplatelet agents on platelet function tests, drug interactions with cART, and clinical data on the reduction of cardiovascular events. While antiretroviral therapy has significantly improved outcomes for people living with HIV, the challenge of the presence of viral reservoirs and drug resistance necessitates innovative new approaches. In addition, poor patient adherence has affected access and impacted quality of care.

This section further discusses new drug options for the future. Gene therapy, discussed in Chapter 3, is the most promising tool for the ultimate cure of infection. The chapter explores the fundamental principles and techniques of gene therapy and highlights the special challenges posed by HIV. It discusses various gene therapy strategies, including gene editing technologies and gene transfer methods, along with their potential advantages and limitations. It also examines safety, efficacy, and ethical concerns in gene therapy for HIV. The chapter urges for strong and continued research within the framework of robust interdisciplinary collaboration. The aim is to inspire further exploration and harnessing of gene therapy's transformative potential in the quest for an HIV cure.

Chapter 4 discusses obesity as an emerging public health problem among people living with HIV/AIDS. It provides an overview of the pathophysiology, impact, and management of obesity within the context of HIV infection, highlighting the most recent advances in this field. The chapter examines the pathophysiology and the pharmacological complex mechanisms by which antiretroviral drugs lead to obesity pathogenesis. Proposed recent mechanisms at the molecular level include improved tolerability, direct impact on adipogenesis, and gut microbiome disturbances. The chapter reviews obesity on a global scale and demonstrates the increasing magnitude in HIV/AIDS patients. The chapter further discusses the treatment of obesity, reviewing its management within the context of a multidisciplinary approach including lifestyle modifications, behavioral therapy, and pharmacotherapy. It also discusses bariatric surgery to address severe obesity. The chapter also highlights new drugs for the treatment of obesity. For instance, orlistat is the sole anti-obesity drug approved; Naltrexone-bupropion may also revolutionize obesity treatment. Other drugs in the pipeline include retatrutide, liraglutide, and semaglutide. Bariatric surgery is gaining popularity as the most effective surgical option to address severe obesity and metabolic dysregulation when lifestyle changes fail to achieve weight goals.

Section three discusses immune reconstitution inflammatory syndrome (IRIS), defined as a clinically significant exacerbation of known low-symptomatic often infectious diseases, which emerge in response to highly active antiretroviral therapy (HAART). It examines how successful HAART treatment leads to a resurgence of known, previously asymptomatic diseases. For example, tuberculosis, both pulmonary and extrapulmonary, occurs very commonly following successful treatment with HAART. Other conditions to a lesser degree but with a similar pathogenesis include leprosy, fungal infections, cryptococcal infection, toxoplasmosis, shingles, and lymphomas.

Chapter 5 examines the pathogenesis of IRIS with special reference to lymphomas, focusing on Hodgkin's lymphoma (HL). HL is considered within the framework of this problem. Unlike other malignant lymphoid tumors that occur with low levels of CD4+ T-lymphocytes, HL develops with elevated levels of CD4+ lymphocytes in response to HAART in HIV-infected patients in the first months of starting antiretroviral treatment. HL was diagnosed in 8% of HIV-infected individuals without HAART. It is revealed that after the administration of HAART, the frequency of HL increased to 17%. This chapter examines these data and discusses the critical role of HAART in the etiology and pathogenesis of HL in HIV-infected patients.

This book contains valuable knowledge and experience from experts worldwide. I thank the authors for their contributions. I also thank Author Service Manager Karmen Daleta at IntechOpen for the valuable support and assistance.

Samuel Okware Ph.D.
Busitema University,
Mbale, Uganda

Section 1

Introduction

Chapter 1

Introductory Chapter: New Emerging Treatment Options for HIV-AIDS

Samuel Okware

1. Introduction

The last three decades HIV/AIDS (human immunodeficiency virus/acquired immunodeficient syndrome) have seen a severe tragedy with worldwide implications on health, society and development. The World Health Organization (WHO) estimated that there were 38 million people living with HIV/AIDS (PLWA), of whom 6.9 million had died. Despite the global efforts, there were about 1.7 million new infections by 2021. Combination antiretroviral therapy (ART) has made significantly positive impact on the lives of people living with HIV/AIDS (PLWA). The ART has reduced mortality significantly and improved wellness and longevity. Trends in new HIV infections have been declining partly due to the test-and-treat strategy using ART that led to viral load suppression and reduced the risk of HIV transmission. Some of these drugs are also used for pre-exposure prophylaxis (PrEP) against HIV infection. Sexual transmission remains the major route of transmission. HIV destroys the immune system, leaving the host susceptible and vulnerable to a variety of bacteria, viruses, fungi and protozoa. Despite global efforts, only 70% infected persons access treatment [1]. Various classes of these drugs are currently available. They include the nucleotide reverse transcriptase inhibitors (NRTI), non-nucleotide reverse transcriptase inhibitors (NNTRI), integrase inhibitors and the protease inhibitors. The combination ART blocks the replication processes, the reverse transcription, protein maturation and the viral integration processes and subsequently inhibits pathways in the HIV life cycle.

2. Challenges in drug treatment

The major drawback of the treatment is the short life and inability to reach potential reservoirs of infection, especially the central nervous system (CNS), lymph nodes, and the lungs and others including latently infected cells, CD4+ T-cells and monocytes. Monocytes are short-lived circulating immune cells that are a precursor to macrophages and immune cells [2]. Increasing the dosage sometimes leads to toxicity. Drug toxicity leads to poor adherence and subsequent drug resistance, noncommunicable diseases and comorbidities. Liver disease is a major drug-induced toxicity and accounts for 13% of deaths in PLWHA [2]. Cardiovascular disease and metabolic disturbances are associated particularly with first-generation drugs, especially Efavirenz and protease inhibitors and Tenofovir, which causes renal damage.

IntechOpen

The other challenge of the treatment is failure to eliminate the integrated proviral genomes in the host cells of individuals with viral suppression. The lifelong treatment involves daily intake of several pills that impact adherence leading to resistance. These limitations have necessitated the exploration of safer and user-friendly drug options for the elimination of the virus to control rebound of viremia once drugs are stopped. Drug-to-drug interactions occasionally occur with oral medications, but very rarely with injectables. Discontinuation of all the antivirals should be avoided, despite the shortcomings.

3. Gene-based therapies

The interest in gene-based therapy arose following the eradication of HIV in the so-called "Berlin patient" who received stem cell transplant from a C-C chemokine receptor type 5 (CCR5) negative donor but who was naturally resistant to human immunodeficiency virus type 1 (HIV1). This single case study demonstrated that complete remission and cure is possible. During the 12th International AIDS Society (IAS) Conference in Brisbane in 2023, it was again demonstrated that the CCR5-targeted gene editing may provide a cure for PLWHA. Mutations at this level block the CCR5 receptor and prevent HIV infection of cluster of differentiation 4 (CD4) T-cells [3]. Thus, infected individuals who are heterozygous for the CCR5 delta 32 mutated gene have slower rates of disease progression. Studies to establish efficacy of the CCR5 inhibitors such as Maraviroc may produce a new class of drugs for HIV/AIDS.

Vaccine approaches aiming at the immune system and through induction of broadly autologous neutralizing antibodies are promising options. Several immune therapies are being developed and tested. This concept if successful will impact significantly on the HIV elimination and contribute to the control of reservoirs. These options could include immune stimulators, immunomodulators and immunotherapies being developed. Vaccine strategies hold the promise for future treatment. The challenges in developing an HIV vaccine are the ability of the virus to mutate and evade the body's immune defenses. The different subvariants may require us to suggest combining different variants into a single vaccine or a combination into a mosaic-based regimen, but there have been several failures including the AIDSVAX trials and the HIV Vaccine Trials Network (HVTN) 505 in 2013 and the HVTN 702 in 2020. The mosaic vaccine approach provides a broader immune response and was demonstrated in the mosaic adenovirus serotype 26 vector (Ad26) vaccine [4]. However, attention should be paid to immune-related severe adverse effects including autoimmunity. Future treatment priorities should focus on gene-based therapies, vaccines, nanotechnology and long-acting injectable regimens to overcome resistance, eliminate reservoirs and promote user-friendly access of interventions [5].

Gene-based technologies and therapies are expanding to new tools for the effective inhibition and precise targeting of the HIV in the body. The clustered regularly interspaced short palindromic repeats (CRISPR)-associated protein-9 nuclease (Cas9) has evolved as an effective genome editing tool that provides the total inhibition of viral replication without the need for long-term continuous treatment. The CRISPR/Cas9 gene-based approaches effectively eradicate HIV-1 by targeting the integrated provirus and eliminate the reservoirs, thus making HIV cure a reality to promote a healthy life without reemergence of infections [6].

4. Nanotechnology-based drugs

The shorter period of availability of these medications in the bloodstream and poor access to targeted tissues remains a challenge. However, nanotechnology has the potential to respond to these issues and deliver antiretroviral (ARV) to treat HIV/AIDS. Nanosystems are structured nanodrug carriers. There are five major nano systems that can be applied for HIV drug entrapment. These include the liposomes, dendrimers, polymeric nanoparticles and solid lipid nanoparticles and inorganic nanoparticle systems. Nanobiotechnologies offer improved performance for manufacturing ART drugs and revolutionizing delivery methods. Nanoparticles are small colloidal particles within the range of 10–100 nm. Nanosystems encase and carry the drug and deliver it by controlling its absorption, distribution, degradation and excretion based on the physical and chemical charges present in the nanotools. These systems have the ability to increase the drug biodistribution and bioavailability and expose the virus particle more precisely for a longer period. Furthermore, these drugs can be delivered directly at the anatomical reservoir site inaccessible by routine drugs.

Nanocarriers can address the therapeutic limitations of current drugs including drug delivery, bioavailability and physicochemical stability. Zidovudine, for instance, is an amphiphilic drug, which when loaded into liposomes resulted in major improvements in distribution in reticuloendothelial system and brain organs and a longer half-life than analog zidovudine. This approach reduced toxicity and improved efficacy. Studies conducted by trapping ARV drugs, such as acyclovir, indinavir, zidovudine and lamivudine into the liposomal structure, demonstrate a 12-fold increase of the drug in blood plasma compared with conventional drugs [7].

Dendrimer formulation nanosystems targeting have also been shown to inhibit the replication of HIV infections. These nanoimmunoliposomes display greater and longer antiviral efficacy than free drugs. The inorganic class of nanoparticle tools contains metal elements such as iron, gold, silver, titanium and silica. Silver nanoparticles, for instance, are becoming more common due to their antimicrobial and antiviral effects.

5. Overcoming resistance

New treatments are emerging to mitigate drug resistance in patients not responding to ART. These drugs will target the persistent multiple drug resistance in PLWHA. Some of these drugs are undergoing clinical trials and include Fostemsavir, Ibalizumab and Lenacapavir. They are still in development stages and were recently approved for experimental use for adults with limited drug options. Fostemsavir is a GP 120 attachment inhibitor and is administered orally twice a day. Ibalizumab's mechanism of action is based on a CD 4-directed postattachment inhibitor. It can be administered intravenously every 2 weeks. Lenacapavir is a capsid inhibitor and can be given subcutaneously every 6 months with an initial oral loading dose. These drugs are promising for patients failing on multiple ART drug regimens. These emerging options can reduce toxicities resulting from other different regimens as well as drug interactions and address patient's socioeconomic preference [8].

Vaccine approaches aim at the induction of broadly autologous neutralizing antibodies that may contribute to reservoir control and are in experimental stages. These efforts include immune stimulators, immunomodulators or agonists and immunotherapies under development.

6. Long-acting ART injectables

Long-term technologies are also emerging as options for PLWHA failing on current contemporary regimens for HIV treatment and prevention. Pre-exposure prophylaxis is a major biomedical tool for HIV prevention. Countries are expanding their HIV prevention strategies by adding dapivirine vaginal ring (DVR) and long-acting injectable Cabotegravir (CAB-LA). A range of other opportunities are being introduced. However, low ART adherence has undermined the strategy for the elimination of HIV infection. Specifically among adolescents and young adults aged 15–24 years, the adherence is unacceptably low. The daily administration of pills often leads to fatigue and frustration. PLWHA has significant barriers, especially among the young people. Such constraints impede timely access to treatment. For instance, complacency, stigma, drug stockouts and side effects are the major obstacles impacting adherence. Other factors include the pill burden, distance from clinic, alcohol and drug abuse. These barriers have persisted at personal and public level and hinder effective service delivery among the youths. For this group, long-acting injectables have been found to be superior and preferred over daily pills.

Injectable Cabotegravir given every 2 months by far is the ideal choice for pre-exposure prophylaxis. This option is a game changer in Africa and other low resource settings. This will target adolescent and young women who are currently very vulnerable key populations [9]. Long-acting injectables can improve adherence among these groups. The ART injections reduce dose frequency and the pill burden and the stigma associated with daily medication. Studies have shown that Cabotegravir injection is highly effective and when administered once every 2 months it was the preferred option over the daily pill. The HPTN 084 trial demonstrated a high preference of 78% compared with taking the pills. Thus, this long- acting injectable intervention presents a real opportunity for scaling up uptake for PrEP.

Thus, Cabotegravir injection is user-friendly and ideal for the young women and adolescents in Africa and countries with low uptake oral PrEP. Youth-friendly services, such as timing and appropriate communication, are needed to overcome the associated barriers. Such communication should be gender sensitive and emphasize patient-centered interface.

7. Conclusion

More antiretroviral therapy (ART) options are emerging for permanent treatment of PLWHA. Future research priorities should be directed at determining the sources and characteristics of the replication of the virus and the link between the cellular reservoirs, the residual plasma viremia and the resistant viruses so as to develop tools to reverse latency. Gene therapy technologies, new vaccine options and long-acting injectable regimens offer the best promise for the elimination of HIV infection. This undertaking should be cognizant of the social, behavioral and ethical research, which aspects should be integrated into HIV clinical trials. Equally important are the impending consequences of aging and upward trends of noncommunicable diseases. The arising inequities in social amenities associated with treatment need to be addressed. Therefore, future HIV programs should integrate social inclusion needs such as jobs, housing and social welfare to support the aging population with comorbidities.

DOI: http://dx.doi.org/10.5772/intechopen.112955

Author details

Samuel Okware[1,2]

1 Uganda National Health Research Organisation, Entebbe, Uganda

2 Busitema University, Mbale, Uganda

*Address all correspondence to: okwares@gmail.com

References

[1] UNAIDS. Global HIV and AIDS Statistics - Fact Sheet 2022, U. Editor. Geneva: UNAIDS; 2022

[2] Veenhuis RT et al. Monocyte-derived macrophages contain persistent latent HIV reservoirs. Nature Microbiology. 2023. DOI: 10.1038/s41564-023-01349-3

[3] Sáez-Cirión AEA. Absence of viral rebound for 20 months without antiretrovirals after allogeneic hematopoietic stem cell transplantation with wild-type CCR5 donor cells to treat a biphenotypic sarcoma abstract OALBA0504. 2023. p. 12

[4] Barough D. Evaluation of a mosaic HIV1 (APPROACH) in rhesus monkeys. Lancet. 2018;**392**:232-243

[5] Deeks SG, Archin N, Cannon P, et al. Research priorities for an HIV cure: International AIDS society global scientific strategy. Nature Medicine. 2021;**27**(12):2085-2098

[6] Bhowmik R. Chaubey CRISPR/Cas9: A tool to eradicate HIV-1 REVIEW. AIDS Research and Therapy. 2022;**19**(58)

[7] Kumar L, Verma S, Prasad DN, Bhardwaj A, Vaidya B, Jain. Nanotechnology: A magic bullet for HIV AIDS treatment. Artificial Cells, Nanomedicine, and Biotechnology. 2015;**43**(2):71-86

[8] Molina J. ClinicalTrials.Gov. Doravirine/Islatravir (DOR/ISL) in heavily treatment-experienced (HTE) participants for human immunodeficiency virus type 1 (HIV-1) infection (MK-8591A-019). In: Abstract OALX01LB02, IAS 2021. Montreal; 2021

[9] Lendevite R. Long acting injection preferred over daily pills for PrEP. AIDS. 2020. PrEP. Availabel from: https://www.cdc.gov/hiv/basics/prep/paying-for-prep/index.html

Section 2

Treatment Considerations for HIV – What's New

Chapter 2

Emerging Clinical Problem of Resistance to Antiplatelet Therapy in Primary Prevention and Treatment of Cardiovascular Events in People Living with HIV: Conundrum despite Effective cART

Gordon Ogweno and Edwin Kimathi

Abstract

Despite the extensive use of combined antiretroviral therapy (cART) for effective human immunodeficiency viral (HIV) suppression, people living with HIV have an increased risk of cardiovascular events compared to the general population. Antiplatelet agents are recommended for primary prevention and treatment of individuals at risk of ischaemic stroke and heart attack. However, these guidelines and recommendations are hinged on data from non-HIV populations. Accumulating evidence has revealed that response to antiplatelet agents varies in people living with HIV compared to non-HIV individuals. The variability may be attributed to consequences of HIV infection, metabolic derangements, and effects of cART and other drug interactions. Given that interventions employed in primary and secondary prevention of cardiovascular events heavily rely on guidelines developed for the general population that emphasize on identification, optimization and stratification of traditional risk factors, there is need to tailor these interventions with knowledge of HIV status and co-administration of cART. This chapter will synthesize the current topic regarding antiplatelet agents in people living with HIV. Specifically, we will critically examine the effects of individual antiplatelet agents on platelet function tests, drug interactions with cart and clinical data on the reduction of cardiovascular events.

Keywords: HIV, antiplatelet therapy, cardiovascular events, treatment, prevention

1. Introduction

Global statistics indicate that 28.7 of the 38.4 million people were living with HIV (PLWH) infection in 2022, 650,000 were on antiretroviral medications and 650,000 deaths were recorded [1]. The availability of effective combined antiretroviral therapy (cART) for HIV infection has transformed the disease from an infectious to a noncommunicable disease (NCD) including cardiovascular events, consisting of aggregate of interrelated chronic conditions, such as chronic inflammation, immune activation and metabolic syndrome (MetS).

The prevalence of MetS among PLWH is high, ranging from 11 to 45% [2] plausibly linked to some cART regimens containing zidovudine, some non-nucleoside reverse transcriptase inhibitor drugs (NNRTIs) (e.g. efavirenz) and protease inhibitors (PIs) (e.g. indinavir) [3, 4]. MetS is a risk factor and precursor for the development of cardiovascular disease [5], in the background of chronic inflammatory processes linked to cardiovascular events [6]. Collectively, these factors combine to aggravate an already existing or accelerate the development of cardiometabolic complications such as intravascular thrombosis.

Platelet hyperactivity links HIV, MetS and cardiovascular diseases [7], and antiplatelet medications are indicated depending on risk stratification in order to prevent cardiovascular complications. However, in the general population, the protective effect of aspirin is variable, with some individuals being resistant [8]. Emerging evidence indicates that the suboptimal response may be greater in PLWH. It is now acknowledged that the risk factors for the development of MetS also modulate the efficacy of antiplatelet agents, resulting in abrogated protection against cardiovascular complications, a phenomenon known as treatment failure or drug resistance.

2. Cardiovascular events in HIV

2.1 Epidemiology of cardiovascular events in HIV

People living with HIV have 50% increased risk of cardiovascular events than non-HIV patients [9] or twofold risk than the general population [10]. Although cardiovascular diseases account for 8–22% deaths among HIV-infected patients, the rates are expected to increase with the aging HIV-infected population on effective cART [11]. Whereas the substantial risk of death associated with HIV infection increases with the use of cART [12], HIV and cART independently exhibit hyperactive platelets in spite of viral suppression [13].

2.2 Ischaemic stroke in HIV

The incidence of ischaemic stroke in HIV is one and half times greater than in non-HIV-positive patients, a situation that persists independently after controlling for other traditional risk factors [14]. The rates are higher across gender and age groups, although younger age groups are more affected in HIV than in non-HIV-infected controls [15]. Hyperactive platelets have been implicated in the independent causal relationship between ischaemic stroke, HIV infection and cART treatment [16]. Surprisingly, the incidence and risk factors are not reduced by cART [17].

3. Antiplatelet therapy in HIV

3.1 Available antiplatelet agents

Available antiplatelet agents fall into various chemical groups acting on different pharmacological targets. Aspirin or acetylsalicylic acid (ASA) at low doses

(30–150 mg) irreversibly blocks constitutive isoenzyme cyclooxygenase-1 (COX-1) in platelets preventing the generation of Thromboxane A2 (TXA2) from membrane arachidonic acid (AA), thus attenuating amplification pathways in platelet activation and aggregation [18]. Given that aspirin acts exclusively *via* arachidonic acid pathway, other signaling pathways stimulated by adenosine diphosphate (ADP), thrombin, collagen, adrenaline and thrombin receptor activating peptide (TRAP) are unaffected. Clopidogrel is an oral thienopyrimidine prodrug that undergoes a series of biotransformation in the hepatic circulation to the active form. It binds selectively and irreversibly to the purinergic receptor P2Y12 on the platelet membrane, blocking access to the platelet agonist ADP [18]. The glycoprotein IIbIIIa (GPIIbIIIa) agents are only available as intravenous (iv) formulations for peri-procedural usage and

Agent	Drug class	Molecular target	Route	Time to onset of action	Time to platelet function recovery after stopping
Aspirin	Acetylsalicylic acid	Irreversible cyclooxygenase 1 (COX-1) inhibition	Oral	20 min	5–7 days
Clopidogrel Ticlopidine Prasugrel	Thienopyridines	Irreversible P2Y12 receptor inhibition	Oral	2–6 h 30 min 30 min	7 days 7–10 days
Cangrelor	Nucleoside/ Nucleotide analogues-Adenosine triphosphate (ATP) analogue	Reversible P2Y12 ADP receptor inhibition	IV	<5 min	30–50 min
Ticagrelor	Nucleoside/ Nucleotide analogues-Cyclopentyl-triazolo-pyrimidine		Oral		3–5 days
Abciximab Eptifibatide Tirofiban	Monoclonal antibody Synthetic RGD analogues	GPIIbIIIa receptor inhibitors	IV	10–20 min	4–8 h
Vorapaxar	Tricyclic himbacine derivative	PAR 1 receptor inhibitor	Oral		4–8 weeks
Cilostazol Dipiridamole	2-Oxoquinoline pyrimidopyridine	PDE-enzyme inhibitor	Oral		12–16 h
Iloprost Beraprost Treprostinil prostacyclin		Prostaglandin (PGI2) analogues	IV/ Inhalation		2 h

Table 1.
Classification of antiplatelet agents, route of administration and time to platelet recovery after cessation.

thereafter replaced by orally available agents for continued long-term antiplatelet therapy (**Table 1**, Antiplatelet agents adapted from [19, 20]).

3.2 Antiplatelet therapy rationale in HIV

People living with HIV (PLWH) have 1.5 times increased risk of cardiovascular events [21] associated with platelet activation exhibiting increased membrane expression of P-selectin [22–24], integrin GPIIbIIIa (PAC-1) [24], microparticles [22] and platelet-leucocyte aggregates [25]. Increased platelet activation and aggregation parameters do not improve with cART treatment [26, 27]. These parameters have been reported as definitive contributors to microvascular thrombosis in heart attack and ischaemic stroke [28] that necessitate antiplatelet therapy [9], especially in sub-Saharan Africa where HIV is most prevalent [29]. The criteria for initiation of antiplatelet therapy in primary prevention of cardiovascular diseases are based on the Framingham risk score [30] that incorporates age (>45 year males, >50 year females) and MetS features [31]. PLWH meet criteria for antiplatelet therapy, though at a much younger age compared to non-HIV [32].

3.3 Antiplatelet therapy and platelet function in HIV

Although aspirin is the most popular and widely used antiplatelet agent, in cART-stabilized HIV patients, an aspirin loading dose of 325 mg oral aspirin followed by a daily oral dose of 81 mg for 5 days failed to suppress urinary and serum thromboxane levels and arachidonic acid (AA)-stimulated Light Transmission Aggregometry (LTA) compared to controls [33]. However, in the same patients, there was a decrease in response to other agonists [33]. The lack of response to aspirin on AA stimulation is consistent with the development of acquired aspirin resistance [34]. This finding contrasts with that of another study where the subjects who received 100 mg oral aspirin for 2 weeks had suppressed urinary and serum thromboxane B2 (TxB2) levels and showed a decrease in AA-stimulated platelets on LTA, surface expression of biomarkers and prolongation of platelet function analyzer-100 (PFA-100) closure time [35], suggesting that the resistance could be overcome by dose increment.

In the Evaluation of Residual Platelet Reactivity After Acute Coronary Syndrome (ST+/ST−) in HIV (EVERE$_2$ST-HIV) study, a comparison of the platelet function in acute coronary syndrome patients on dual antiplatelet therapy (a combination of aspirin and P2Y12 inhibitors) found that the proportion of patients with residual platelet reactivity for both drugs was higher in HIV + ve patients compared to non-HIV, as assessed by residual platelet aggregation (RPA) on LTA, platelet reaction units (PRUs) on VerifyNow and platelet reaction index (PRI) on vasodilator-associated protein (VASP) [13]. In the same study, the resistance showed to antiplatelet remedies was consistent across the drugs and the methods of assay, correlated with HIV status but was greater with protease inhibitors more than NNRT [13].

The EVERE$_2$ST-HIV study findings demonstrated that platelet reactivity is high among patients with recurrent acute coronary syndrome and that antiplatelet therapy was associated with: (i) high residual platelet reactivity on a number of laboratory tests, (ii) resistance displayed to aspirin, clopidogrel, prasugrel and ticagrel, (iii) resistance was correlated with HIV RNA viral load, cluster of differentiation 4 (CD4) count and cART, and (v) genetic polymorphism was uniformly distributed across all study groups and therefore could not account for drug responses [13]. The observed high value on treatment with the antiplatelet agents could provide an explanation for recurrent ischaemic events in PLWH.

Another study that evaluated aspirin, clopidogrel and placebo on platelets in PLWH reported interesting findings summarized as follows: (i) diminished platelet aggregation upon aspirin administration on LTA stimulated by arachidonic acid and ADP, even though the platelet receptor expression evaluated by flow cytometry remained unaffected; (ii) clopidogrel lowered ADP (but not AA)-induced platelet aggregation on LTA and showed greater suppression of platelet activation biomarkers (P-selectin, PAC-1) and (iii) clopidogrel, but not aspirin, decreased endothelial and inflammatory biomarkers after 2 weeks of treatment compared to aspirin or placebo [36]. The results of this study suggested that suboptimal response may be limited to aspirin, and clopidogrel may provide a better profile and therefore may be the preferred therapy in PLWH. The uncoupling of responses between aggregation and activation and differences in drug responses indicate that aspirin inhibition of COX-1 does not protect against platelet hyperactivity from HIV-associated immune activation consistent with other studies [37].

Overall, the studies on PLWH suggest that platelet resistance to aspirin is higher compared to clopidogrel and potentially illustrates that platelet activation is not solely dependent on COX-1. Although data point to aspirin resistance in HIV, it must be noted that PLWH present with preexisting platelet hyperactivity prior to initiation of antiplatelet therapy [33]. Aspirin inhibition of platelet functions is selective for arachidonic acid-stimulated pathway, but insensitive to other agonists [38]. Consequently, this suggests that the application of cut-off levels to test results may be inappropriate to categorize patients, given the variability to aspirin response in normal individuals with pre-existing platelet hyperactivity [39].

3.4 Clinical thrombosis and antiplatelet therapy in HIV

Despite adequate antiplatelet therapy and other interventions during the first episode of acute coronary thrombosis, high recurrence rates still continue to be reported in HIV patients [40, 41]. This observation therefore indicates clinical resistance to antiplatelet medication in PLWH. However, the clinical spectrum and mechanisms have not been well defined.

3.5 Other outcomes of antiplatelet therapy in HIV

Aspirin's potential to dampen the inflammatory response has been employed for the treatment of an array of inflammatory conditions over the years [42, 43]. On this basis, a clinical trial pilot study in stable cART-treated patients found that the administration of a 325 mg oral loading dose of aspirin followed by 81 mg daily decreased T-cell activation (cluster of differentiation 38 (CD38) and human leucocyte antigen-DR (HLA-DR)) and monocyte activation (soluble cluster of differentiation 13 (CD13)), but enhanced leucocyte response to toll-like receptor (TLR) stimulation [33], suggestive of attenuation of immune responses. Similarly, in another study, 81 mg aspirin reduced T-cell activation and genital mucosal inflammation in PLWH [44]. However, a clinical trial by the same investigators comparing 300 mg and 100 mg aspirin with placebo over a 12-week period did not reveal any difference in inflammatory markers such as soluble cluster of differentiation 14 (CD14), interleukin 6 (IL-6), cluster of differentiation 163 (CD163), T-cell activation or any other inflammatory markers [37], indicating that cardioprotective doses of aspirin have no effect on inflammation. Consistent with other studies, administration of low-dose aspirin (81 mg) in premature coronary artery disease (CAD) over 14 days failed to lower elevated inflammatory markers such as high-sensitivity C-reactive protein (hs-CRP) and IL-6 whose levels correlated with urinary 11-dehydrothromboxane B2 (uTxM), biomarker of aspirin resistance [45]. Moreover, low-dose aspirin in HIV patients does not attenuate pro-inflammatory lipid mediators of inflammation [46].

4. Concept and mechanism of antiplatelet resistance

4.1 Concept of antiplatelet resistance

The concept of antiplatelet resistance encompasses a variety of broad phenomena such as suboptimal, poor or nonresponse, treatment failure or variability. In the narrowest sense, it refers specifically to endogenous mechanism in certain individuals, which prevents the drug from exerting its full antithrombotic effect when applied at therapeutic doses compared to expectations in normal individuals [47–50]. It is multifactorial and includes both clinical and laboratory evidence of deficiency in activity, despite adequate therapy and compliance. The incidence varies widely in studies depending on the antiplatelet agent, methodology of assessment and cut-off levels.

Clinical 'resistance' to antiplatelet drugs has been defined to occur with the onset of new, or worsening of ischaemic cardiovascular events in particular in patients while on recommended appropriate doses of antiplatelet agents. It is broad and encompasses treatment failure, interindividual variability or failure to protect from thrombotic ischaemic vascular events. Since this terminology does not imply the cause-effect relationship between the presence of drug and consequent events, its use is discouraged [18].

Chemical or true resistance specifically refers to de-acetylation of cyclooxygenase 1 at serine 529 (COX-1 Ser529) in platelets by aspirin. There are no chemical definitions of Thienpyrimidines or GPIIbIIIa blockers' resistance. Individuals resistant to clopidogrel are grouped into intermediate or poor metabolizers. Intermediate metabolizers process some clopidogrel, so they receive partially benefit from the treatment but are not protected from developing a harmful blood clot. Poor metabolizers process little or no clopidogrel, so they benefit minimally from the treatment and are at risk of forming a harmful blood clot.

Laboratory 'resistance' to antiplatelet drugs refers to lack of, poor response, nonresponsiveness or deficiency of platelet reactivity on *in vitro* tests, despite the use of oral antiplatelet drugs when evaluated on a predetermined cut-off level of inhibition [18]. This pharmacological definition refers to the lack of effect at the target site of action upon stimulation by agonist specific to each drug on the various platelet function tests. It may, or may not be specific to inhibition of a COX-1 system. Based on pharmacokinetic and pharmacodynamic characteristics, laboratory resistance has been stratified into three levels [51, 52], namely:

i. Responders: Normal platelet aggregation and TxB2 levels >95.2 ng/ml. Therapeutic oral aspirin blocks platelet aggregation and reduces TxB2 to <0.5 ng/ml.

ii. Type I resistance: Pharmacokinetic, reduced bioavailability at sites of action. *Ex vivo* platelet aggregation is not inhibited and TxB2 levels ≤82.9 ng/ml. TxB2 levels and platelet aggregation are successfully inhibited by *in vitro*-added antiplatelet agents.

DOI: http://dx.doi.org/10.5772/intechopen.112500

iii. Type II resistance: Pharmacodynamic, normal bioavailability at sites of action. Platelet aggregation is present, but TxB2 is partially reduced to ≤32–17 ng/ml by oral aspirin. Persistent TxA2 is present in serum and urine due to altered sites of action. Thromboxane A2 and platelet aggregation takes place when antiplatelet is added *in vitro*. Accelerated platelet turnover takes place, with introduction into bloodstream of newly formed, drug unaffected platelets. It is suggestive of COX-1 inhibition with persistent platelet activation, possibly from inducible cyclooxygenase 2 (COX-2) production of prostaglandin H2 (PGH2) conversion to TXA2, increased sensitivity to other agonists such as ADP, epinephrine, collagen and thrombin.

iv. Type III resistance: pseudo-resistance or treatment failure. Oral aspirin does not inhibit platelet aggregation but Thromboxane A2 is successfully inhibited by both *in vivo* and *in vitro* added antiplatelet agents. Platelet aggregation can cause to be inhibited from non-TXA2-mediated pathways, such as due to smoking, hypercholesterolaemia, exercise or stress.

Because the different antiplatelet drugs block different pharmacological targets, it has been proposed that aspirin resistance be restricted to COX-1-dependent TXA-2 pathways, while that of thienopyrimidine (clopidogrel) be limited to the inability to inhibit purinergic P2Y12 receptor pathways [48]. There is evidence to suggest that resistance occurs to direct GPIIbIIIa inhibitors [53] but data are limited.

4.2 Laboratory measurement of antiplatelet resistance

The laboratory methods, in definition of antiplatelet resistance, involve either biochemical or functional assays. Due to the complexity in relating clinical outcomes to laboratory tests, and the performance and interpretation of test results, a consensus statement that guides the testing of aspirin resistance has been compiled by a group of experts [54]. In summary, they recommend as prerequisites that include the following points: the patient needs to be on stable antiplatelet therapy for at least 5 days and there should be confirmation of compliance and method for establishing drug bioavailability either in plasma or urine.

The recommended tests are a combination of biochemical (urinary or serum TXA2) and functional (platelet aggregation-LTA) assays. The assays should include *in vitro* addition of COX-1 inhibitor (aspirin) and COX-2 inhibitor if necessary to further elucidate the mechanism. Analysis of membrane surface receptor expression may be performed to characterize polymorphisms.

4.2.1 Bleeding time (BT)

This is the oldest method for the assessment of primary hemostasis that demonstrated the prolongation of bleeding time (BT) with ingestion of aspirin [55, 56]. In a clinical trial of aspirin, a subset of healthy volunteers (40%) and patients undergoing coronary artery bypass graft (CABG) (42%) were nonresponders as therapeutic doses of aspirin failed to prolong bleeding time [57]. In other studies, bleeding time of nonresponders [58] correlated with alternative *in vitro* platelet function test [59]. However, there is great unpredictability in responses ranging from exaggerated (increased bleeding time) response [59] to paradoxical prothrombotic (decreased) bleeding time in some individuals [60] or lack of correlation with other laboratory tests [61].

4.2.2 The biochemical assays

4.2.2.1 COX-1-dependent assay

During platelet activation, arachidonic acid is metabolized to intermediate prostaglandins in reactions catalyzed by COX-1 mainly, and COX-2 under special conditions. The terminal end products, thromboxane metabolites, are stable and appear in urine and serum. Thus, the measurement of TxA2 metabolite (serum thromboxane-A2) and urinary 11-dehydrothromboxane-B2 (11dhTxB2) [62] reveals activation status. Low-dose aspirin (30–300 mg) specifically blocks the COX-1 pathway leading to low activation sates (low serum/urine thromboxane metabolites). As urine levels of TxB2 usually vary depending on the rate and volume of urine collected, no normal values have been agreed upon [63]. Owing to this, it is recommended that the urinary TXB2 be correlated with creatinine levels, such that nonresponders have TxB2 > 33.8 ng/mmol cr while levels in partial responders are 15.1 to 33.8 ng/mmol cr [64]. The results are influenced by non-COX-1 sources of TxA2 that include thromboxane synthases in monocytes, macrophages and endothelial cells. Furthermore, COX-2 can also produce TxA2 independent of COX-1 [62]. Although aspirin consistently suppresses platelet COX-1 production of thromboxanes in platelets, there is lack of uniformity upon evaluation by functional assays [65].

4.2.2.2 Intraplatelet VASP assay

Vasodilator-stimulated phosphoprotein (VASP) is an intracellular protein whose activity links purinergic P2Y12 receptor occupancy to intracellular signaling leading to GPIIbIIIa activation with attendant fibrinogen binding [66]. During platelet activation, ADP occupancy of platelet P2Y12 receptors leads to VASP dephosphorylation, GPIIbIIIa activation and fibrinogen binding. Conversely, clopidogrel displacement of ADP at P2Y12 receptors triggers VASP phosphorylation (VASP-P) and stabilizes GPIIbIIIa in an inactive resting state that cannot bind fibrinogen [67, 68]. Thus, assays of intracellular VASP-P (flow cytometry or enzyme-linked immunosorbent assay (ELISA)) can estimate the level of platelet inhibition by thienopyrimidine (such as clopidogrel). Platelet VAS-P assay results are presented as platelet reactivity index (PRI) [69]. Since high levels of VASP-P correspond to low PRI [67, 70], there is an almost linear inverse relationship between PRI and level of P2Y12 blockade [68]. Because of the latter relationship, VASP is considered a specific biomarker for thienopyrimidine (e.g. clopidogrel) on purinergic P2Y12-mediated pathways, although it does not indicate the extent of receptor activation or aggregation.

4.2.3 Platelet functional assays

The commonly used clinical platelet functional assays include:

4.2.3.1 Platelet aggregometry

i. Light transmission aggregometry (LTA): It is considered the gold standard reference for platelet function testing stratifying aspirin responders as Aspirin sensitive (AS) or Aspirin resistant (AR). Of the various agonists used, AA has high specificity as it amplifies COX-1 synthesis of TxA2 targeted by aspirin. The cut-off for AR is agonist and dose dependent, but consensus considers the AA concentration at 1.6 mg/mL as appropriate for the investigation of AR [62].

ii. Platelet function analyzer-100 (PFA-100™): It consists of passage of whole blood through capillary apertures coated with a combination of either collagen or ADP (Coll/ADP) or collagen and epinephrine (Coll/Epi). When platelets are stimulated with either epinephrine or ADP, they plug the aperture and time to closure (CT) is recorded. Aspirin prolongs the closure time beyond 300 s. It is considered specific for aspirin.

iii. VerifyNow™ system: It is a whole blood-based turbidometric method where blood is passed through cartridges coated with a combination of fibrinogen and agonists for pathways to be t-tested for each drug, as in AA for aspirin, TRAP for GPIIbIIIa inhibitors and ADP or PGE1 to be tested for each drug, such that AA for aspirin, TRAP for GPIIbIIIa inhibitors and ADP or PGE1 for purinergic P2Y12 receptor blockers. In this assay, changes in light transmittance correspond to level of platelet aggregation. Platelet adhesion occurs in proportion to available fibrinogen receptors and results reported in aspirin response (aspirin reaction unit (ARU)), the normal value being >550 [64]. It was developed to monitor aspirin effects on platelets.

Test	Agonist	Cut-off	ASA cut-off [71]	Clopidogrel cut-off [71]
VerifyNow [62]	ADP, AA, TRAP	PRU > 208	ARU > 550	>240 clopidogrel reaction units
Biochemical serum and urine TxA2 [62]	—	AR urine >1500 pg./mg cr Serum >3.1 ng/mg cr	Urine 11dhTxB2 > 67.9 ng/mmol cr	
MEA [62]	ADP, AA, TRAP, collagen	AU > 46 AR > 30%		
TEG platelet mapping	ADP	Ma > 47 mm		
VASP	PGE1 and ADP	PRI > 50%		N > 70 PRI Clo > 50%PRI
RPFA [64]	Cationic propyl thiogallate	ARU > 550		
PFA-100 [62, 64]	Coll/ADP (CADP) Coll/Epinephrine (CEPI)	CT > (N < 163–190 s) CADP <(69–140 s) CEPI< (80–200 s)	CT(N < 193)	
LTA [62, 72]	AA (0.5–1 mg/mL) ADP (10 μmol/L)	≥20% AA ≥70ADP ≥70%collagen	>20%	<10% reduction
TEG [72]	Platelet mapping	≥50%AA		
P-selectin [73]	Flow cytometry	+ve cells>5%		
GPIIbIIIa [74]	Flow cytometry	Log MFI > 220		

Table 2.
Laboratory tests in the evaluation of antiplatelet resistance and their cut-off levels.

iv. Impedance aggregometry (Multiple electrical aggregometry-MEA™/Multiplate): Impedance aggregometry (Multiple electrical aggregometry-MEA™/Multiplate) uses whole blood sample to measure change in electrical resistance as platelets are activated by agonists. The results are expressed in ohms (Ω) or Area under the curve (AUC) calculated from aggregation units (AUs) after subtracting baseline levels obtained with 0.9% saline (**Table 2**).

4.2.4 Flow cytometry

The method uses monoclonal antibodies to identify and quantify platelets' membrane receptor expression of P-selectin (alpha granule secretion), GPIIbIIIa or fibrinogen binding (PAC-1), glycoprotein Ib-V-IX (GPIb-V-IX) and CD40 ligand (CD40L). These antibodies are used to characterize the extent of pharmacogenetic influence on antiplatelet resistance in combination with gene profiling [75]. Notably, P-selectin expression is less sensitive to aspirin effects in patients [76], as opposed to healthy volunteers [77]. More importantly, patients who require antiplatelet agents, such as for acute coronary syndrome and ischaemic stroke, already have preexisting increased platelet expression that is not abrogated by aspirin or clopidogrel [78]; thus, it is a less sensitive indicator of antiplatelet resistance.

4.2.5 Global coagulation assays

Thromboelastography (TEG) estimates platelet functions in whole blood in the presence of other cellular elements including red blood cells (RBCs) and leucocytes thus considered more physiological. A modified technique, platelet mapping, defines the contribution of platelets to clot strength using AA or ADP. In comparison with other tests, it is less precise [79] and overestimates platelet resistance [80].

4.2.6 Comparison of methods

Generally, near-patient testing methods, such as PFA-100, VerifyNow™ and Impedance Aggregometry, are preferred for clinical testing [81]. Since antiplatelet drugs block diverse signaling pathways, the recommended agonists for pathways testing include AA for aspirin and ADP for thienopyrimidine (e.g. clopidogrel) [82]. While it has been observed that platelets are resistant to aspirin, they exhibit hypersensitivity to low dose or submaximal doses of agonists on a dose-response curve [83].

While it is generally agreed that some individuals exhibit suboptimal response to antiplatelet medication, there is no consensus on laboratory investigation since various methods have been employed. Similarly, there is disagreement on the interpretation of laboratory test results that report increased platelet activation during treatment and linkage to clinical events for clinical decision-making is still debatable [84]. Many clinicians prefer the term 'high on treatment platelet reactivity' [85], equivalent to decreased effectiveness [86]. High on treatment platelet reactivity (HTPR) is a screening tool to estimate platelet functions while on treatment. However, the various methods give different incidence/prevalence values of aspirin resistance. Furthermore, when compared to each other, there is wide heterogeneity and lack of concordance with biochemical tests and therefore are not interchangeable [87]). Notably, optical aggregometry (LTA), VerifyNow and PFA-100 each gives different values for the prevalence of aspirin resistance in patients with ischaemic stroke [88]. However, they neither showed reproducibility nor correlation/agreement with one another [79]. Overall, the available evidence shows that TEG-PM is least suitable [80], whereas Multiplatelet Impedance method serves as the most reproducible, acceptable reliable method among healthy donors and patients for monitoring antiplatelet medications [80]. Moreover, test results vary on a temporal scale depending on the timing of blood collection from the onset of treatment [80]. Given that drug responses follow a bell-shaped curve, the interindividual responses on the platelet function tests could plausibly be a reflection of normal biological distribution on either side of the curve but not true resistance [80]. The differences in responses could arise from alternative activation pathways not targeted by the drugs tested [80].

4.3 Mechanisms of antiplatelet resistance

Factors contributing to the resistance mechanisms arise from changes at the clinical, cellular and genetic levels [89]. In the case for aspirin, the mechanisms are characterized as Thromboxane dependent or independent, while the diverse clopidogrel mechanisms encompass genetic polymorphism of purinergic receptors. The modulating factors act at the level of pharmacokinetic/pharmacodynamic resistance, platelet properties, postreceptor signaling and metabolic conditions such as diabetes mellitus, insulin sensitivity and obesity [64].

Pharmacokinetic resistance occurs when, despite ingestion of adequate doses of aspirin, there is failure of inhibition of COX-1 owing to inadequate plasma levels, malabsorption or genetic polymorphism [90]. Pharmacodynamic resistance is experienced when thromboxane production continues despite adequate COX-1 inhibition, due to COX-2 from other sources [90]. Pseudo-resistance is characterized by the total inhibition of thromboxane but platelet activation still occurs through thromboxane-independent pathways such as ADP, epinephrine or thrombin [90].

The proposed biological basis for aspirin resistance [91] includes the following points: (i) aspirin-insensitive TxA2 biosynthetic pathways *via* inducible COX-2 or regenerated COX-1 from other cells such as macrophages, monocytes and endothelium; (ii) alternate platelet activation pathways arising from increased sensitivity to collagen, catecholamine surges (exercise, stress), non-TxA2-mediated (e.g. ADP, thrombin and platelet activating factor (PAF)); (iii) prostaglandin-like compounds (lipid peroxidation); and (iv) vascular inflammation due to increased expression of CD40L.

4.4 Management of antiplatelet resistance

Although there is a growing body of evidence regarding resistance to antiplatelet agents in the general population and in PLWH in particular, no consensus has been formed on the appropriate laboratory method to detect it, or whether laboratory evaluation should be routinely performed in clinical practice. Furthermore, it is still unclear whether treatment failures are due to drug resistance, or how the drug resistance results translate to clinical outcomes. Queries regarding PLWH on antiplatelet therapy have been raised (on whether the right agents are being used either singly or in combination) [92]. Nevertheless, the general practice is to increase the dosage, while balancing against the risk of adverse drug effects, especially gastrointestinal (GI) bleeding. Alternatively, adding another antiplatelet (dual therapy), which acts through a different pathway, may be an option [93]. Alternatively, a switch to another agent with less resistance, or adding a third antiplatelet agent, may be considered.

5. Risk factors for antiplatelet resistance in HIV

5.1 cART interactions as contributors to antiplatelet resistance in HIV

Human immunodeficiency viral infection and some cART contribute to platelet hyperactivity [94]. In the EVERE$_2$ST-HIV study, patients receiving cART with PIs and other combinations had increased platelet reactivity to P2Y12 inhibitors and higher prevalence of HPR, consistent across all functional tests (RPA, VASP-PRI and PRU). Conversely, patients treated with NNRTIs had consistently decreased platelet reactivity and lower prevalence of HPR [95]. According to this study, resistance was consistent for aspirin across all cART, but variable for P2Y12 inhibitors.

In other studies (e.g. ATP-binding cassette (ABC)-treated patients) though, aspirin reduced urinary and serum Thromboxane A2 and AA induced platelet aggregation on LTA, indicating treatment compliance. Other biomarkers remain above cut-off levels of reactivity and did not normalize compared to healthy uninfected controls [35], indicating suboptimal response or resistance to therapy.

The mechanism of cART-induced platelet hyperreactivity includes induction of MetS [96] and modulation of extra-platelet enzymatic degradation of nucleotides promoting feedback activation by ADP [97]. cART also contributes to suboptimal antiplatelet effects through pharmacokinetic drug interactions. PIs and NNRTIs are strong inhibitors of hepatic cytochrome P450 3A (CYP3A) enzymes, diminish clopidogrel and prasugrel bioactivation and decrease the bioavailability of the active drug metabolite, thereby decreasing antiplatelet effects [92, 98].

5.2 Other concomitant drug (proton pump inhibitor (PPI), statins, antifungals and over-the-counter nonsteroidal anti-inflammatory drugs (OTC NSAIDs) interactions and antiplatelet resistance in HIV

There is potential for drug interactions in PLWH, owing to the intake of multiple drugs.

Many PLWH are on proton pump inhibitors (PPIs) for bleeding prophylaxis or to counteract the effects of antiplatelet or nonsteroidal anti-inflammatory drugs (NSAIDs). Coronary artery disease (CAD) patients treated with daily oral 75 mg aspirin together with PPI exhibit increased platelet aggregation than those not on PPI [99], indicating suboptimal response to aspirin. Similarly, omeprazole decreases antiplatelet effects of clopidogrel as evaluated by VASP PRI [100]. Clinically, patients on aspirin or clopidogrel plus PPI have increased incidence of major adverse cardiovascular events [101, 102]. By acting on platelet cyclooxygenase, over-the-counter treatment (OTC) NSAIDs displace aspirin from its active site, thus decreasing its effectiveness [103].

5.3 Concomitant infections and antiplatelet resistance in HIV

Concomitant bacterial, viral, fungal and mycobacterial (e.g. tuberculosis) infections are common in PLWH. Early in sepsis, platelet activation and aggregation are enhanced compared to healthy controls with variation in levels observed between Gram-positive and Gram-negative bacteria [104, 105]. Whereas agonist-induced aggregation deteriorates with progression of sepsis severity [106–109], activation biomarkers as demonstrated by the expression of adhesion molecules (cluster of differentiation 42a (CD42a), cluster of differentiation 42b (CD42b), cluster of differentiation 36 (CD36), cluster of differentiation 29 (CD29) and PAR-1) [110] and alpha granule secretion (P-selectin) [105, 111] remain unchanged, or increased [112]. However, when platelet count is taken into account, aggregation and activation status correlate [113] with the overall phenomenon of increase in platelet reactivity with sepsis severity [114]. Microorganisms and their products such as lipopolysaccharides interact with platelets directly through TLR, and indirectly *via* bridging proteins that include fibrinogen, fibronectin, von Willebrandt factor (vWF) and thrombospondin through platelet receptors such as GPIIbIIIa and GPIa-IX-V [115].

5.4 Metabolic syndrome/hyperlipidaemia complications and antiplatelet resistance in HIV

Metabolic syndrome (MetS), characterized by insulin resistance, visceral adiposity, atherogenic dyslipidaemia and endothelial dysfunction [31], occurs in PLWH partly due to HIV, and due to some cART [2, 116]. The prevalence of MetS in PLWH could be as high as 21% [3]. MetS is associated with exaggerated platelet function [117] and the suboptimal response to aspirin in up to 69% patients [118–120]. The decreased response to aspirin in MetS may be due to hyperlipidaemia, inflammation (high hs-CRP) [121] and increased platelet turnover that releases large reticulocytes into circulation [122] with enhanced expression of COX-2 [123] being less sensitive to aspirin [124, 125]. Furthermore, apoptotic platelet changes induced by HIV [126], hyperlipidaemia [127] and aspirin [128] mimic laboratory characteristics of antiplatelet resistance. The independent factor contributing to platelet hyperactivity in MetS appears to have increased hs-CRP, a marker of inflammation [129].

5.5 Deficiencies of vitamin D and other micronutrients as risk factors for antiplatelet resistance in HIV

Vitamin D deficiency is a common finding in HIV infection [130, 131]. The said deficiency is associated with platelet activation [132] and antiplatelet resistance [133]. In vitamin D deficiency, platelet hyperactivity is triggered by oxidative stress [134] and immune activation [135, 136]. These factors increase MetS-linked endothelial activation [137] and cause platelet-endothelial adhesive protein vWF release [138] leading to activation via GPIb-IX-V receptors by bypassing the aspirin-inhibited pathway, thus enhancing the risk of thrombosis.

Magnesium contributes to antiplatelet effects [139, 140] by: (i) interfering with fibrinogen binding of GPIIbIIIa due to induced membrane alterations, (ii) competing with membrane transporters of Ca++, and (iii) intracellular signal transduction pathways that promote Ca++ influx and mobilization from stores [140, 141] (e) decreasing thromboxane biosynthesis [142, 143]. Also, hypomagnesaemia produces oxidative stress and increased risk of cardiovascular events [144].

Although diet has not been specifically investigated in relation to antiplatelet resistance in HIV, there is strong justification for its contribution as a risk factor. Diets rich in micronutrients and vitamins, such as practiced among Mediterranean population, are reputed to lower cardiovascular risk factors due to antiplatelet effects [145]. It is speculated that individuals who do not partake these diets may be at risk of micronutrient deficiencies and rebound platelet hyperactivity.

5.6 Inflammation, megakaryopoiesis/reticulated platelets in HIV

Human immunodeficiency viral (HIV) infection is characterized by high levels of inflammation. Elevated inflammatory biomarkers, such as hs-CRP, tumor necrosis factor α (TNF-α) and phospholipase 2 (PLA2), are associated with platelet hyperactivity and aspirin resistance [146–148]. Inflammation contributes to aspirin resistance through several mechanisms including initiation of COX-1-independent platelet activation mechanisms, acceleration of platelet turnover and thrombopoiesis, generation of reticulated platelets rich in COX-2, generation of reactive oxygen species (ROS) and promotion of the expression of surface adhesion molecules, such as P-selectin, GPIIbIIIa and CD40L [89]. vWF, a platelet-vascular adhesive molecule released during inflammation [149], is a biomarker elevated in HIV [150, 151]. It contributes to aspirin resistance [146] through platelet activation via glycoprotein Ib (GPIb) receptor [152]. The signaling pathways are independent of COX-1-mediated thromboxane. Immune complexes and complements bind to platelets and activate platelets through immunoreceptor tyrosine-based activation motif (ITAM) signaling pathways [153, 154].

People living with HIV have enhanced megakaryopoiesis characterized by increased immature platelet reticulocytes in circulation (up to 10%) compared to control non-HIV [155, 156]. Although immature platelets display increased agonist-stimulated aggregation and membrane activation receptor expression [157], these responses persist, despite antiplatelet therapy [125], consistent with resistance to medication. Antiplatelet resistance arises due to increased expression of COX-2 during maturation [158] that is neither inhibited by aspirin nor inhibited by clopidogrel [124].

5.7 Gut microbial translocation and platelet hyperactivity in HIV

HIV virus is highly predisposed to localize in the gut epithelial lining, and CD4 and CD8 (cluster of differentiation 8) lymphocytes in underlying Peyer's patches and lymph nodes. The subsequent epithelial destruction leads to loss of barrier functions, resulting in 'leaky gut' and passage of gut microbiota into the systemic circulation, a process termed 'gut microbial translocation' [159]. The translocated bacteria, and their products, such as lipopolysaccharides (LPS) and Trimethylamine N -oxide (TMAO), interact with platelet Toll-like receptor-4 (TLR-4) contributing to platelet hyperactivity [160]. Although it has been demonstrated that in non-HIV, acute coronary patients with translocated gut microbiota have platelet hyperactivity despite being on antiplatelet agent ticagrelor [161], no data on antiplatelet resistance are available for PLWH.

5.8 Racial and genetic polymorphisms in antiplatelet resistance and HIV

People of African descent have higher rates of vascular ischaemic events compared to other racial groups, a phenomenon that persists even after the administration of antiplatelet medications [162]. Genetic polymorphism disaggregated based on race arises in response to antiplatelet medications [163]. African Americans exhibit clopidogrel HTPR as assessed on VerifyNow (PRU) and VASP (PRI) compared to Caucasians, which corresponds to a higher prevalence of CYP2C19*2 allele carrier status [164]. The response is also reflected in LTA and VerifyNow testing patients on aspirin and clopidogrel at baseline and on stimulation with other agonists at different concentrations [165]. The differences could be traced to genetic polymorphism to GPIIbIIIa and P2Y12 receptors [166]. Plausibly, genetic polymorphism could explain the antiplatelet resistance reported in a study of PLWH where a majority of them were people of black ancestry [36]. However, it must be emphasized that although data suggest that the people of African descent are likely more resistant to antiplatelets compared to other races, the reality is that less than one fifth of those who qualify for and could potentially benefit actually are prescribed for and take antiplatelets [167].

6. Guidelines for antiplatelet therapy

6.1 Guidelines for antiplatelet therapy in HIV

Globally, incidences of noncommunicable diseases (NCDs) are on the rise [168], partly due to HIV infection [169]. For the primary prevention of cardiovascular events, the US Preventive Task Force (USPTF) recommends the calculation of risk assessment and initiation of antiplatelet therapy to those who meet the criteria [170]. Despite the unique risk factors for cardiovascular events in HIV [32], no specific guidelines exist for antiplatelet therapy for HIV-specific cardiovascular preventive strategies, despite the concerns raised [171]. Unfortunately, many guidelines have not incorporated focused antiplatelet therapy for at-risk PLWH, despite thrombosis being reported in many case series in patients not on aspirin [172]. Despite the known cardiovascular risks in HIV, antiplatelets are grossly underutilized in PLWH [173–175]. Even in centres where antiplatelets are prescribed, disparities in prescription and quality of care are rampant [176], resulting in high rates of adverse cardiovascular events among PLWH [177]. Whereas the potential for drug-to-drug interactions between cART and antiplatelets is real, a study found aspirin and clopidogrel dual therapy continues to be prescribed alongside PI and NNRTI in coronary artery disease, resulting in 100% adverse interactions [92].

6.2 Guidelines for laboratory testing of antiplatelet resistance

Although it is clear that antiplatelet resistance is glaring, most professional societies' guidelines do not consider that there is sufficient evidence to routinely perform the laboratory evaluation of antiplatelet resistance to justify altering prescribing practice based on platelet function testing results [62]. The role of routine aspirin or any other antiplatelet therapy in primary prevention of cardiovascular events is increasingly being questioned, since it only targets 25% of cardiovascular events, the rest being from other causes [178]. Thus, the emergence of drug resistance or suboptimal response introduces a new dimension in the conundrum of care for cardiovascular diseases in general, and HIV in particular. Given the escalating burden of cardiovascular diseases, and the role of platelets in pathophysiology, there is a burgeoning paradigm shift away from the traditional approach of risk stratification, antiplatelet therapy and platelet function testing for research purposes. The current direction is a personalized approach, whereby individual platelet phenotypes are evaluated by alternative means and targeting therapy [179]. Currently, it is increasingly becoming clear that there is a lack of equipoise in testing and therapeutic practice, instead, further studies are recommended to guide practice.

7. Conclusion

The incidence of major cardiovascular events, including acute coronary syndromes and ischaemic stroke, is elevated in PLWH and hyperactive platelets are implicated. The risk factors for hyperactive platelets include HIV, cART and the attendant metabolic syndrome. Although guidelines recommend antiplatelets such as aspirin, the problem of their resistance in HIV is greater than in the general population, which predisposes to greater morbidity and mortality risk. Identification of drug resistance in laboratory functional assays is challenging, owing to the different definitions of the phenomenon and the limitations of correlating it with clinical observations. It is emerging that the contributing factors to platelet hyperactivity and related antiplatelet drug (e.g. aspirin) resistance are the interplay of concurrent inflammation, micronutrient deficiencies and drug interactions acting at both pharmacokinetic and pharmacodynamic levels. Although many guidelines have been developed for antiplatelet medications in cardiovascular disease management, none is specific for HIV. Despite effective uptake of cART globally, the issue of antiplatelet medication in PLWH is a conundrum. The population most affected by HIV and concurrent MetS who meet the criteria for antiplatelet medications are not getting it. The reasons are unclear, but may include the lack of awareness and screening for MetS, not following the guidelines with regard to problems in polypharmacy. Even in cases where antiplatelets are prescribed, the emergence of antiplatelet resistance hampers effective primary prevention or treatment of cardiovascular events in PLWH.

Author details

Gordon Ogweno[1*] and Edwin Kimathi[2]

1 Department of Medical Physiology, Kenyatta University, Nairobi, Kenya

2 Department of Medical Biochemistry, Kisii University, Kisii, Kenya

*Address all correspondence to: ogweno.gordon@ku.ac.ke

References

[1] UNAIDS. Global HIV statistics. Fact Sheet. 2022;**2022**:1-6

[2] Paula AA, Falcão MCN, Pacheco AG. Metabolic syndrome in HIV-infected individuals: Underlying mechanisms and epidemiological aspects. AIDS Research and Therapy. 2013;**10**(1):32. DOI: 10.1186/1742-6405-10-32

[3] Todowede OO, Mianda SZ, Sartorius B. Prevalence of metabolic syndrome among HIV-positive and HIV-negative populations in sub-Saharan Africa—A systematic review and meta-analysis. Systematic Reviews. 2019;**8**(1):1-17. DOI: 10.1186/s13643-018-0927-y

[4] Rwegerera GM et al. Metabolic control and determinants among hiv-infected type 2 diabetes mellitus patients attending a tertiary clinic in Botswana. Diabetes, Metabolic Syndrome and Obesity. 2021;**14**:85-97. DOI: 10.2147/DMSO.S285720

[5] Guembe MJ et al. Risk for cardiovascular disease associated with metabolic syndrome and its components: A 13-year prospective study in the RIVANA cohort. Cardiovascular Diabetology. 2020;**19**(1):1-14. DOI: 10.1186/s12933-020-01166-6

[6] Sukumaran L et al. Association between inflammatory biomarker profiles and cardiovascular risk in individuals with and without HIV. AIDS. 2023;**37**(4):595-603. DOI: 10.1097/QAD.0000000000003462

[7] Santilli F, Vazzana N, Liani R, Guagnano MT, Davì G. Platelet activation in obesity and metabolic syndrome. Obesity Reviews. 2012;**13**(3):27-42. DOI: 10.1111/j.1467-789X.2011.00930.x

[8] Gum PA, Kottke-Marchant K, Welsh PA, White J, Topol EJ. A prospective, blinded determination of the natural history of aspirin resistance among stable patients with cardiovascular disease. Journal of the American College of Cardiology. 2003;**41**(6):961-965. DOI: 10.1016/S0735-1097(02)03014-0

[9] Boccara F et al. HIV and coronary heart disease: Time for a better understanding. Journal of the American College of Cardiology. 2013;**61**(5):511-523. DOI: 10.1016/j.jacc.2012.06.063

[10] Boccara F, Cohen A. HIV and heart disease: What cardiologists should know. Revista Española de Cardiología (English Edition). 2016;**69**(12):1126-1130. DOI: 10.1016/j.rec.2016.05.032

[11] Seecheran VK, Giddings SL, Seecheran NA. Acute coronary syndromes in patients with HIV. Coronary Artery Disease. 2017;**28**(2):166-172. DOI: 10.1097/MCA.0000000000000450

[12] D'Ascenzo F et al. Acute coronary syndromes in human immunodeficiency virus patients: A meta-analysis investigating adverse event rates and the role of antiretroviral therapy. European Heart Journal. 2012;**33**(7):875-880. DOI: 10.1093/eurheartj/ehr456

[13] Hauguel-Moreau M et al. Platelet reactivity in human immunodeficiency virus infected patients on dual antiplatelet therapy for an acute coronary syndrome: The EVERE2ST-HIV study. European Heart Journal. 2017;**38**(21):1676-1686. DOI: 10.1093/eurheartj/ehw583

[14] Chow FC, Regan S, Feske S, Meigs JB, Grinspoon SK, Triant VA.

Comparison of ischemic stroke incidence in HIV-infected and non-HIV-infected patients in a US health care system. Journal of Acquired Immune Deficiency Syndromes. 2012;**60**(4):351-358. DOI: 10.1097/QAI.0b013e31825c7f24

[15] Schaefer JH, Stephan C, Foerch C, Pfeilschifter W. Ischemic stroke in human immunodeficiency virus-positive patients: An increasingly age-related comorbidity? European Stroke Journal. 2020;**5**(3):252-261. DOI: 10.1177/2396987320927672

[16] Benjamin LA et al. HIV infection and stroke : Current perspectives and future directions. Lancet Neurology. 2012;**11**(10):878-890. DOI: 10.1016/S1474-4422(12)70205-3

[17] Landrø L, Ueland T, Otterdal K, Frøland SS, Aukrust P. Persistently raised plasma levels of platelet-derived inflammatory mediators in HIV-infected patients during highly active anti-retroviral therapy. Journal of Thrombosis and Haemostasis. 2011;**9**(5):1075-1077. DOI: 10.1111/j.1538-7836.2011.04242.x

[18] Kuliczkowski W et al. Interindividual variability in the response to oral antiplatelet drugs: A position paper of the working group on antiplatelet drugs resistance appointed by the section of cardiovascular interventions of the polish cardiac society, endorsed by the working. European Heart Journal. 2009;**30**(4):426-435. DOI: 10.1093/eurheartj/ehn562

[19] Michelson AD. Antiplatelet therapies for the treatment of cardiovascular disease. Nature Reviews. Drug Discovery. 2010;**9**(2):154-169. DOI: 10.1038/nrd2957

[20] Jourdi G, Godier A, Lordkipanidzé M, Marquis-Gravel G, Gaussem P. Antiplatelet therapy for Atherothrombotic disease in 2022—From population to patient-centered approaches. Frontiers in Cardiovascular Medicine. 2022;**9**(January):1-19. DOI: 10.3389/fcvm.2022.805525

[21] Freiberg MS et al. HIV infection and the risk of acute myocardial infarction. JAMA Internal Medicine. 2013;**173**(8):614-622. DOI: 10.1001/jamainternmed.2013.3728

[22] Mayne E et al. Increased platelet and microparticle activation in HIV infection : Upregulation of P-selectin and tissue factor expression. Journal of Acquired Immune Deficiency Syndromes. 2012;**59**(4):340-346

[23] Nkambule BB, Davison G, Ipp H. The value of flow cytometry in the measurement of platelet activation and aggregation in human immunodeficiency virus infection. Platelets. 2015;**26**(3):250-257. DOI: 10.3109/09537104.2014.90909021

[24] Marcantoni E et al. Platelet transcriptome pro fi ling in as a mediator of platelet activity. Journal of the American College of Cardiology: Basic to Translational Science. 2018;**3**(1):9-22. DOI: 10.1016/j.jacbts.2017.10.005

[25] Nkambule BB, Davison G, Ipp H. Platelet leukocyte aggregates and markers of platelet aggregation, immune activation and disease progression in HIV infected treatment naive asymptomatic individuals. Journal of Thrombosis and Thrombolysis. 2015;**40**(4):458-467. DOI: 10.1007/s11239-015-1212-8

[26] O'Halloran JA et al. The effect of initiation of antiretroviral therapy on monocyte, endothelial and platelet function in HIV-1 infection. HIV Medicine. 2015;**16**(10):608-619. DOI: 10.1111/hiv.12270

[27] Taylor KA et al. Pharmacological impact of antiretroviral therapy on

platelet function to investigate human immunodeficiency virus—Associated cardiovascular risk. British Journal of Pharmacology. 2019;**176**:879-889. DOI: 10.1111/bph.14589

[28] Gurbel PA, Defilippi CR, Bliden KP, Tantry US. HIV infection, ACS, PCI and high platelet reactivity: Ingredients for a perfect thrombotic storm. European Heart Journal. 2017;**38**(21):1687-1689. DOI: 10.1093/eurheartj/ehw630

[29] Bloomfield GS, Velazquez EJ. Hiv and cardiovascular disease in sub-saharan africa: The Sutton law as applied to global health. JACC. 2013;**61**(23):2391-2396. DOI: 10.1016/j.jacc.2013.02.041

[30] Tornero C, Ventura A, Mafe M. Aspirin is indicated for primary prevention of cardiovascular events in HIV-infected patients evaluation of the safety of Nevirapine therapy during pregnancy. Journal of Acquired Immune Deficiency Syndromes. 2010;**54**(5):560-567

[31] Huang PL. A comprehensive definition for metabolic syndrome. Disease Models & Mechanisms. 2009;**2**(5-6):231-237. DOI: 10.1242/dmm.001180

[32] Feinstein MJ et al. Characteristics, prevention, and Management of Cardiovascular Disease in people living with HIV: A scientific statement from the American Heart Association. Circulation. 2019;**140**(2):e98-e124. DOI: 10.1161/CIR.0000000000000695

[33] O'Brien M et al. Aspirin attenuates platelet activation and immune activation in HIV-1-infected subjects on antiretroviral therapy: A pilot study. Journal of Acquired Immune Deficiency Syndromes. 2013;**63**(3):280-288. DOI: 10.1097/QAI.0b013e31828a292c

[34] Krishnan K, Nguyen TN, Appleton JP, Law ZK, Caulfied M, Cabrera CP, et al. Antiplatelet resistance : A review of concepts , mechanisms , and implications and transient ischemic attack. Stroke: Vascular and Interventional Neurology. 2023;**0**:e000576. DOI: 10.1161/SVIN.122.000576

[35] Falcinelli E et al. Effect of aspirin treatment on abacavir-associated platelet hyperreactivity in HIV-infected patients. International Journal of Cardiology. 2018;**263**(2017):118-124. DOI: 10.1016/j.ijcard.2018.04.052

[36] Marcantoni E et al. Antiplatelet effects of Clopidogrel vs aspirin in Virologically controlled HIV. A randomized controlled trial. JACC Basic to Translational Science. 2022;**7**(11):1086-1097. DOI: 10.1016/j.jacbts.2022.06.002

[37] O'Brien MPO et al. A randomized placebo controlled trial of aspirin effects on immune activation in chronically human immunodeficiency virus-infected adults on Virologically suppressive antiretroviral therapy. Open Forum Infectious Diseases. 2017;**4**(1):ofw278. DOI: 10.1093/ofid/ofw278

[38] Taylor ML, Ilton MK, Misso NLA, Watkins DN, Hung J, Thompson PJ. The effect of aspirin on thrombin stimulated platelet adhesion receptor expression and the role of neutrophils. British Journal of Clinical Pharmacology. 1998;**46**(2):139-145. DOI: 10.1046/j.1365-2125.1998.00766.x

[39] Frelinger AL et al. Aspirin 'resistance': Role of pre-existent platelet reactivity and correlation between tests. Journal of Thrombosis and Haemostasis. 2008;**6**(12):2035-2044. DOI: 10.1111/j.1538-7836.2008.03184.x

[40] Bravo I, Álvarez H, Mariño A, Clotet B, Moltó J. Recurrent coronary disease in HIV-infected patients: Role

of drug–drug interactions. British Journal of Clinical Pharmacology. 2018;**84**(7):1617-1619. DOI: 10.1111/bcp.13583

[41] Boccara F et al. Acute coronary syndrome in human immunodeficiency virus-infected patients: Characteristics and 1 year prognosis. European Heart Journal. 2011;**32**(1):41-50. DOI: 10.1093/eurheartj/ehq372

[42] Amann R, Peskar BA. Anti-inflammatory effects of aspirin and sodium salicylate. European Journal of Pharmacology. 2002;**447**(1):1-9. DOI: 10.1016/S0014-2999(02)01828-9

[43] Morris T et al. Effects of low-dose aspirin on acute inflammatory responses in humans. Journal of Immunology. 2009;**183**(3):2089-2096. DOI: 10.4049/jimmunol.0900477

[44] Lajoie J, Birse K, Mwangi L, Chen Y, Cheruiyot J, Akolo M. Using safe, affordable and accessible non-steroidal anti-inflammatory drugs to reduce the number of HIV target cells in the blood and at the female genital tract. Journal of the International AIDS Society. 2018;**21**(7):e25150. DOI: 10.1002/jia2.25150

[45] Qayyum R, Faraday N, Yanek LR, Vaidya D, Becker LC, Becker DM. Abstract 5067:Responsiveness to low dose aspirin influences levels of inflammatory biomarkers. Circulation. 2008;**118**(Abstract):S_1138-S_1139

[46] Dalli J et al. Pro-inflammatory and pro-resolving lipid mediators of inflammation in HIV: Effect of aspirin intervention. eBioMedicine. 2023;**89**:1-10. DOI: 10.1016/j.ebiom.2023.104468

[47] Michelson AD, Frelinger AL, Furman MI. Resistance to antiplatelet drugs. European Heart Journal. 2006;**8**(Supplement G):G53-G58. DOI: 10.1093/eurheartj/sul056

[48] Cattaneo M. Resistance to antiplatelet drugs : Molecular mechanisms and laboratory detection. Journal of Thrombosis and Haemostasis. 2007;**5**(Suppl. 1):230-237

[49] Saraf S, Bensalha I, Gorog DA. Antiplatelet resistance — Does it exist and how to measure it ? Clinical Medicine. Cardiology. 2009;**3**:77-91

[50] Mărginean A, Bănescu C, Scridon A, Dobreanu M. Anti-platelet therapy resistance – Concept , mechanisms and platelet function tests in intensive care facilities. Journal of Critical Care Medicine. 2016;**2**(1):6-15. DOI: 10.1515/jccm-2015-0021

[51] Weber AA, Przytulski B, Schanz A, Hohlfeld T, Schrör K. Towards a definition of aspirin resistance: A typological approach. Platelets. 2002;**13**(1):37-40. DOI: 10.1080/09537100120104890

[52] Patel JA, Bhatt DA, Chorawala MR, Deshpande SS, Shah GB. Aspirin Resistance: Molecular Mechanisms & Techniques. IJPRS. 2011;**2**(07):1623-1630

[53] Van Werkum JW et al. Inhibition of platelet function by abciximab or high-dose tirofiban in patients with STEMI undergoing primary PCI: A randomised trial. Netherlands Heart Journal. 2007;**15**(11):375-381. DOI: 10.1007/BF03086018

[54] Pulcinelli FM, Riondino S. More on: Aspirin resistance: Position paper of the working group on aspirin resistance. Proposal for a laboratory test guiding algorithm. Journal of Thrombosis and Haemostasis. 2006;**4**(2):485-487. DOI: 10.1111/j.1538-7836.2006.01755.x

[55] Mielke CH, Kaneshiro MM, Maher IA, Weiner JM, Rapaport SI. The standardized and its normal prolongation ivy bleeding by aspirin time. Blood. 1969;**34**(2):204-216

[56] Amrein PC, Ellman L, Harris WH. Aspirin-induced prolongation of bleeding time and perioperative blood loss. JAMA. 1981;**245**(18):1825-1828

[57] Buchanan MR, Brister SJ. Individual variation in the effects of ASA on platelet function: Implications for the use of ASA clinically. Canadian Journal of Cardiology. 1995;**11**(3):221-227

[58] Maleki A et al. Aspirin resistance in different doses by bleeding time and urinary 11-dehydro-thromboxane B2. Indian Journal of Physiology and Pharmacology. 2016;**60**(1):30-37

[59] Kawasaki T, Ozeki Y, Igawa T, Kambayashi JI. Increased platelet sensitivity to collagen in individuals resistant to low-dose aspirin. Stroke. 2000;**31**(3):591-595. DOI: 10.1161/01.STR.31.3.591

[60] O'Grady J, Moncada S. Aspirin: A paradoxical effect on bleeding-time. Lancet. 1978;**312**(8093):780. DOI: 10.1016/S0140-6736(78)92661-2

[61] Amezcua JL, Salmon JOGJA, Moncada S, Court L, Br K. Prolonged paradoxical effect of aspirin on platelet behaviour and bleeding time in man. Thrombosis Research. 1979;**2**:69-79

[62] Van Oosterom N, Barras M, Cottrell N, Bird R. Platelet function assays for the diagnosis of aspirin resistance. Platelets. 2022;**33**(3):329-338. DOI: 10.1080/09537104.2021.1942816

[63] Grinstein J, Cannon CP. Aspirin resistance : Current status and role of tailored therapy. Clinical Cardiology. 2012;**35**(11):673-681. DOI: 10.1002/clc.22031

[64] Guthikonda S, Lev EI, Kleiman NS. Resistance to antiplatelet therapy. Current Cardiology Reports. 2005;**7**(4):242-248. DOI: 10.1007/s11886-005-0044-0

[65] Santilli F et al. Platelet cyclooxygenase inhibition by low-dose aspirin is not reflected consistently by platelet function assays. Implications for aspirin 'resistance',. Journal of the American College of Cardiology. 2009;**53**(8):667-677. DOI: 10.1016/j.jacc.2008.10.047

[66] Horstrup K, Jablonka B, Hönig-Liedl P, Just M, Kochsiek K, Walter U. Phosphorylation of focal adhesion vasodilator-stimulated phosphoprotein at Ser157 in intact human platelets correlates with fibrinogen receptor inhibition. European Journal of Biochemistry. 1994;**225**(1):21-27. DOI: 10.1111/j.1432-1033.1994.00021.x

[67] Barragan P et al. Resistance to Thienopyridines : Clinical detection of coronary stent thrombosis by monitoring of vasodilator-stimulated phosphoprotein phosphorylation. Catheterization and Cardiovascular Interventions. 2003;**302**(June 2002):295-302. DOI: 10.1002/ccd.10497

[68] Aleil B, Ravanat C, Cazenave JP, Rochoux G, Heitz A, Gachet C. Flow cytometric analysis of intraplatelet VASP phosphorylation for the detection of clopidogrel resistance in patients with ischemic cardiovascular diseases. Journal of Thrombosis and Haemostasis. 2005;**3**(1):85-92. DOI: 10.1111/j.1538-7836.2004.01063.x

[69] Mallouk N, Varvat J, Berger A, Epinat M, Accassat S, Garcin A. Assessment of a fl ow cytometry

technique for studying signaling pathways in platelets: Monitoring of VASP phosphorylation in clinical samples. Practical Laboratory Medicine. 2018;**11**:10-18. DOI: 10.1016/j.plabm.2018.02.002

[70] Schwarz UR, Geiger J, Walter U, Eigenthaler M. Flow cytometry analysis of intracellular VASP phosphorylation for the assessment of activating and inhibitory signal transduction pathways in human platelets. Definition and detection of Ticlopidine/Clopidogrel effects. Thrombosis and Haemostasis. 1999;**82**:1145-1152

[71] Ben-Dor I, Kleiman NS, Lev E. Assessment, mechanisms, and clinical implication of variability in platelet response to aspirin and Clopidogrel therapy. The American Journal of Cardiology. 2009;**104**(2):227-233. DOI: 10.1016/j.amjcard.2009.03.022

[72] Gurbel PA et al. Evaluation of dose-related effects of aspirin on platelet function: Results from the aspirin-induced platelet effect (ASPECT) study. Circulation. 2007;**115**(25):3156-3164. DOI: 10.1161/CIRCULATIONAHA.106.675587

[73] Xu ZH, Jiao JR, Yang R, Luo BY, Wang XF, Wu F. Aspirin resistance: Clinical significance and genetic polymorphism. The Journal of International Medical Research. 2012;**40**(1):282-292. DOI: 10.1177/147323001204000128

[74] Sane DC, Mckee SA, Malinin AI, Serebruany VL. Frequency of aspirin resistance in patients with congestive heart failure treated with antecedent aspirin. The American Journal of Cardiology. 2002;**9149**(02):893-895

[75] Macchi L et al. Resistance in vitro to low-dose aspirin is associated with platelet Pl A1 (GP IIIa) polymorphism but not with C807T (GP Ia/IIa) and C-5T Kozak (GP Ibα) polymorphisms. Journal of the American College of Cardiology. 2003;**42**(6):1115-1119. DOI: 10.1016/S0735-1097(03)00921-5

[76] Hübl W et al. Assessing aspirin-induced attenuation of platelet reactivity by flow cytometry. Thrombosis Research. 2007;**121**(1):135-143. DOI: 10.1016/j.thromres.2007.03.018

[77] Mckenzie ME et al. Aspirin inhibits surface glycoprotein IIb / IIIa , P-selectin, CD63 , and CD107a receptor expression on human platelets. Blood Coagulation & Fibrinolysis. 2003;**14**:249-253. DOI: 10.1097/01.mbc.0000046182.72384.ab

[78] Bath PM, May J, Heptinstall S, Bath PM, May J, Heptinstall S. Clinical utility of remote platelet function measurement using P-selectin : Assessment of aspirin, clopidogrel, and prasugrel and bleeding disorders clinical utility of remote platelet function measurement using P-selectin : Assessment of aspirin, clop. Platelets. 2018;**29**(5):425-430. DOI: 10.1080/09537104.2018.1445839

[79] Gurbel PA et al. Evaluation of dose-related effects of aspirin on results from the aspirin-induced platelet effect (ASPECT) study. Circulation. 2007;**115**:3156-3164. DOI: 10.1161/CIRCULATIONAHA.106.675587

[80] Tantry US, Bliden KP, Gurbel PA. Overestimation of platelet aspirin resistance detection by thrombelastograph platelet mapping and validation by conventional aggregometry using arachidonic acid stimulation. Journal of the American College of Cardiology. 2005;**46**(9):1705-1709. DOI: 10.1016/j.jacc.2005.05.090

[81] Sibbing D et al. Updated expert consensus statement on platelet function and genetic testing for guiding P2Y12 receptor inhibitor treatment in percutaneous coronary intervention. JACC. Cardiovascular Interventions. 2019;**12**(16):1521-1537. DOI: 10.1016/j.jcin.2019.03.034

[82] Michelson AD. Methods for the measurement of platelet function. The American Journal of Cardiology. 2009;**103**(3 SUPPL):20A-26A. DOI: 10.1016/j.amjcard.2008.11.019

[83] Guthikonda S et al. Increased platelet sensitivity among individuals with aspirin resistance—Platelet aggregation to submaximal concentration of arachidonic acid predicts response to antiplatelet therapy. Thrombosis and Haemostasis. 2008;**100**(1):83-89. DOI: 10.1160/TH07-10-0590

[84] Ait-mokhtar O, Bonello L, Benamara S, Paganelli F. High on treatment platelet reactivity. Heart, Lung and Circulation. 2012;**21**(1):12-21. DOI: 10.1016/j.hlc.2011.08.069

[85] Cattaneo M, Paolo OS, Medicina D, Odontoiatria C. Laboratory detection of 'aspirin resistance ': What test should we use (if any)? European Heart Journal. 2007;**28**:1673-1675. DOI: 10.1093/eurheartj/ehm232

[86] Wiśniewski A, Filipska K. The phenomenon of clopidogrel high on-treatment platelet reactivity in ischemic stroke subjects: A Comprehensive Review. International Journal of Molecular Sciences. 2020;**21**(17):6408. DOI: 10.3390/ijms21176408

[87] Lordkipanidzé M, Pharand C, Schampaert E, Turgeon J, Palisaitis DA, Diodati JG. A comparison of six major platelet function tests to determine the prevalence of aspirin resistance in patients with stable coronary artery disease. European Heart Journal. 2007;**28**(14):1702-1708. DOI: 10.1093/eurheartj/ehm226

[88] Harrison P, Segal H, Blasbery K, Furtado C, Silver L, Rothwell PM. Screening for aspirin responsiveness after transient ischemic attack and stroke: Comparison of 2 point-of-care platelet function tests with optical aggregometry. Stroke. 2005;**36**(5):1001-1005. DOI: 10.1161/01.STR.0000162719.11058.bd

[89] Acikel S, Akdemir R. The relationship between inflammation, platelet activation and antiplatelet resistance. Inflammation & Allergy-Drug Targets. 2010;**9**(5):364-381. DOI: 10.2174/187152810793938017

[90] Yaturu S. Biomarkers of aspirin resistance. Recent Patents on Biomarkers. 2012;**3**(1):57-64. DOI: 10.2174/22103090130105

[91] Mason PJ, Jacobs AK, Freedman JE. Aspirin resistance and atherothrombotic disease. Journal of the American College of Cardiology. 2005;**46**(6):986-993. DOI: 10.1016/j.jacc.2004.08.070

[92] Archer O et al. Patients living with HIV and coronary disease: Are we using appropriate anti platelets as part of dual antiplatelet therapy? Cardiology & Vascular Research. 2021;**5**(1):1-5. DOI: 10.33425/2639-8486.1094

[93] Cañivano Petreñas L, García Yubero C. Resistance to aspirin: Prevalence, mechanisms of action and association with thromboembolic events. A narrative review. Farmacia hospitalaria (English Edition). 2010;**34**(1):32-43. DOI: 10.1016/s2173-5085(10)70062-9

[94] Falcinelli E et al. In vivo platelet activation and platelet hyperreactivity in abacavir-treated HIV-infected patients. Thrombosis and Haemostasis. 2013;**110**(2):349-357. DOI: 10.1160/TH12-07-0504

[95] Hauguel-moreau M et al. Platelet reactivity in human immunodeficiency virus infected patients on dual antiplatelet therapy for an acute coronary syndrome : The-HIV study. European Heart Journal. 2017;**38**:1676-1686. DOI: 10.1093/eurheartj/ehw583

[96] Sapuła M, Suchacz M, Załęski A, Wiercińska-Drapało A. Impact of combined antiretroviral therapy on metabolic syndrome components in adult people living with HIV : A literature review. Viruses. 2022;**14**:122. DOI: 10.3390/v14010122

[97] Felipe J et al. ScienceDirect effect of antiretroviral therapy in thromboregulation through the hydrolysis of adenine nucleotides in platelets of HIV patients. Biomedicine & Pharmacotherapy. 2016;**79**:321-328. DOI: 10.1016/j.biopha.2016.02.008

[98] Egan G, Hughes CA, Ackman ML. Drug interactions between antiplatelet or novel Oral anticoagulant medications and antiretroviral medications. The Annals of Pharmacotherapy. 2014;**48**(6):734-740. DOI: 10.1177/1060028014523115

[99] Wurtz M, Grove EL, Kristensen SD, Hvas A. The antiplatelet effect of aspirin is reduced by proton pump inhibitors in patients with coronary artery disease. Heart. 2010;**96**:368-372. DOI: 10.1136/hrt.2009.181107

[100] Gilard M et al. Influence of omeprazole on the antiplatelet action of Clopidogrel associated with aspirin. The randomized, double-blind OCLA (omeprazole CLopidogrel aspirin) study. Journal of the American College of Cardiology. 2008;**51**(3):256-260. DOI: 10.1016/j.jacc.2007.06.064

[101] Hu W, Tong J, Kuang X, Chen W, Liu Z. In fl uence of proton pump inhibitors on clinical outcomes in coronary heart disease patients receiving aspirin and clopidogrel. Medicine (Baltimore). 2018;**97**(3):e9638

[102] Ono M et al. Impact of proton pump inhibitors on efficacy of antiplatelet strategies with ticagrelor or aspirin after percutaneous coronary intervention : Insights from the GLOBAL LEADERS trial. Catheterization and Cardiovascular Interventions. 2022;**100**:72-82. DOI: 10.1002/ccd.30217

[103] Patrono C et al. Clinical pharmacology of platelet cyclooxygenase inhibition. Circulation. 1985;**72**(6):1177-1184

[104] Tunjungputri RN, van de Heijden W, Urbanus RT, de Groot PG, van der Ven A, de Mast Q. Higher platelet reactivity and platelet-monocyte complex formation in gram-positive sepsis compared to gram-negative sepsis. Platelets. 2017;**28**(6):595-601. DOI: 10.1080/09537104.2016.1252837

[105] Vardon-Bounes F et al. Evolution of platelet activation parameters during septic shock in intensive care unit. Platelets. 2022;**33**(6):918-925. DOI: 10.1080/09537104.2021.2007873

[106] Gawaz M, Dickfeld T, Bogner C, Fateh-Moghadam S, Neumann FJ. Platelet function in septic multiple organ dysfunction syndrome. Intensive Care Medicine. 1997;**23**(4):379-385. DOI: 10.1007/s001340050344

[107] Lundahl TH, Petersson J, Fagerberg IH, Berg S, Lindahl TL. Impaired platelet function correlates

with multi-organ dysfunction . A study of patients with sepsis. Platelets. 1998;**9**:223-225

[108] Boldt J, Menges T, Wollbruck M, Sonneborn S, Hempelmann G. Platelet function in critically ill patients. Chest. 1994;**106**(3):899-903. DOI: 10.1378/chest.106.3.899

[109] Woth G et al. Platelet aggregation in severe sepsis. Journal of Thrombosis and Thrombolysis. 2011;**31**(1):6-12. DOI: 10.1007/s11239-010-0486-0

[110] Salat A et al. Changes of platelet surface antigens in patients suffering from abdominal septic shock. Thrombosis Research. 1999;**95**(6):289-294. DOI: 10.1016/S0049-3848(99)00046-8

[111] Yaguchi A, Lobo FLM, Vincent JL, Pradier O. Platelet function in sepsis. Journal of Thrombosis and Haemostasis. 2004;**2**(12):2096-2102. DOI: 10.1111/j.1538-7836.2004.01009.x

[112] Russwurm S et al. Platelet and leukocyte activation correlate with the severity of septic organ dysfunction. Shock. 2002;**17**(4):263-268. DOI: 10.1097/00024382-200204000-00004

[113] Laursen MA, Larsen JB, Larsen KM, Hvas A. Platelet function in patients with septic shock. Thrombosis Research. 2020;**185**(May 2019):33-42. DOI: 10.1016/j.thromres.2019.11.011

[114] Akinosoglou K, Theodoraki S, Xanthopoulou I, Perperis A, Gkavogianni T, Pistiki A. Platelet reactivity in sepsis syndrome: Results from the PRESS study. European Journal of Clinical Microbiology & Infectious Diseases. Official publication of the European Society of Clinical Microbiology. 2017;**36**(12):2503-2512. DOI: 10.1007/s10096-017-3093-6

[115] Hamzeh-cognasse H, Damien P, Chabert A, Pozzetto B, Cognasse F, Garraud O. Platelets and infections – Complex interactions with bacteria. Frontiers in Immunology. 2015;**6**:1-18. DOI: 10.3389/fimmu.2015.00082

[116] Sprenger H. Antiretroviral therapy only partially reverses the. hypercoagulable state and reduced fibrinolytic potential of HIV-1 infection. In: HIV infection and treatment: Beyond viral control. [Thesis fully internal (DIV), University of Groningen]. Rijksuniversiteit Groningen; 2017

[117] Carvalho ACA, Colman RW, Lees RS. Platelet function in hyperproteinemia. The New England Journal of Medicine. 1974;**290**:434-438

[118] Friend M, Vucenik I, Miller M. Platelet responsiveness to aspirin in patients with hyperlipidaemia. BMJ. 2003;**326**(January):82-83

[119] Smith JP et al. Suboptimal inhibition of platelet Cyclooxygenase-1 by aspirin in metabolic syndrome. Hypertension. 2012;**59**:719-725. DOI: 10.1161/HYPERTENSIONAHA.111.181404

[120] Garshick MS, Teresa M, Vivas M, Drenkova K, Berger JS. Platelet aggregation is enhanced in those with metabolic syndrome and incompletely inhibited by aspirin. Journal of the American College of Cardiology. 2023;**81**(8):1817. DOI: 10.1016/S0735-1097(23)02261-1

[121] Kahraman G et al. The frequency of aspirin resistance and its risk factors in patients with metabolic syndrome. International Journal of Cardiology. 2007;**115**:391-396. DOI: 10.1016/j.ijcard.2006.10.025

[122] Singh A et al. Hyperlipidemia and platelet parameters: Two sides of the same coin. Cureus. 2022;**14**(6):10-16. DOI: 10.7759/cureus.25884

[123] Guthikonda S et al. Reticulated platelets and uninhibited COX-1 and COX-2 decrease the antiplatelet effects of aspirin. Journal of Thrombosis and Haemostasis. 2007;**5**(3):490-496. DOI: 10.1111/j.1538-7836.2007.02387.x

[124] Weber AA, Zimmermann KC, Meyer-Kirchrath J, Schrör K. Cyclooxygenase-2 in human platelets as a possible factor in aspirin resistance. Lancet. 1999;**353**(9156):900-901. DOI: 10.1016/S0140-6736(99)00498-5

[125] Guthikonda S et al. Role of reticulated platelets and platelet size heterogeneity on platelet activity after dual antiplatelet therapy with aspirin and Clopidogrel in patients with stable coronary artery disease. Journal of the American College of Cardiology. 2008;**52**(9):743-749. DOI: 10.1016/j.jacc.2008.05.031

[126] Mesquita EC et al. Persistent platelet activation and apoptosis in virologically suppressed HIV-infected individuals. Scientific Reports. 2018;**8**(1):1-10. DOI: 10.1038/s41598-018-33403-0

[127] Sener A, Ozsavci D, Oba R, Demirel GY, Uras F, Yardimci KT. Do platelet apoptosis, activation, aggregation, lipid peroxidation and platelet-leukocyte aggregate formation occur simultaneously in hyperlipidemia? Clinical Biochemistry. 2005;**38**(12):1081-1087. DOI: 10.1016/j.clinbiochem.2005.09.005

[128] Zhao L, Zhang W, Chen M, Zhang J, Zhang M, Dai K. Aspirin induces platelet apoptosis. Platelets. 2013;**24**(8):637-642. DOI: 10.3109/09537104.2012.754417

[129] Kubica A et al. The impact of metabolic syndrome on the antiplatelet effect of clopidogrel and aspirin in patients with acute coronary syndrome. Folia Medica Copernicana. 2014;**2**(2):66-72. Available from: www.fmc.viamedica.pl

[130] Mueller NJ et al. High prevalence of severe vitamin D deficiency in combined antiretroviral therapy-naive and successfully treated Swiss HIV patients. AIDS. 2010;**24**(January):1127-1134. DOI: 10.1097/QAD.0b013e328337b161

[131] Cervero M et al. Higher vitamin D levels in HIV-infected out-patients on treatment with boosted protease inhibitor monotherapy. HIV Medicine. 2013;**14**(April):556-562. DOI: 10.1111/hiv.12049

[132] Surmen S, Ozer PK, Emet S, Govdeli EA, Elitok A. Biomarkers association between multiplate-measured aspirin resistance and vitamin D deficiency in stable coronary artery disease. Archives of Medical Science - Atherosclerotic Diseases. 2021;**6**:e203-e208. DOI: 10.5114/amsad.2021.112242

[133] Lu B, Shi X, Liang L, Dong N, Liu Z. Platelet surface CD62p and serum vitamin D levels are associated with Clopidogrel resistance in Chinese patients with ischemic stroke. Journal of Stroke and Cerebrovascular Diseases. 2019;**28**(5):1323-1328. DOI: 10.1016/j.jstrokecerebrovasdis.2019.01.031

[134] Oliveira SR, Alfieri DF, Ueda LT, Dichi I, Reiche EMV. Association between vitamin D status , oxidative stress biomarkers and viral load in human immunodeficiency virus type 1 infection. Current HIV Research. 2017;**15**:1-9. DOI: 10.2174/1570162X15666171005170227

[135] Blondon M et al. Associations of serum 25-hydroxyvitamin d with hemostatic and inflammatory biomarkers in the multi-ethnic study of atherosclerosis. The Journal of Clinical Endocrinology and Metabolism. 2016;**101**(6):2348-2357. DOI: 10.1210/jc.2016-1368

[136] Jiménez-sousa MÁ, Martínez I, Medrano LM. Vitamin D in human immunodeficiency virus infection: Influence on immunity and disease. Frontiers in Immunology. 2018;**9**(458):00458. DOI: 10.3389/fimmu.2018.00458

[137] Tabrizi R, Akbari M, Lankarani KB, Heydari ST, Kolahdooz F. The Effects of Vitamin D Supplementation on Endothelial Activation among Patients with Metabolic Syndrome and Related Disorders: A Systematic Review and Meta-Analysis of Randomized Controlled Trials. Nutrition & metabolism. 2018;**15**:85. DOI: 10.1186/s12986-018-0320-9

[138] Cohen-Hagai K et al. Effect of vitamin D status on Von Willebrand factor and ADAMTS13 in diabetic patients on chronic hemodialysis. Annals of Laboratory Medicine. 2017;**37**(2):155-158

[139] Bode C, Gross S, Peter K. The effect of intravenously administered magnesium on platelet function in patients after cardiac surgery. Anesthesia and Analgesia. 1999;**88**:1213-1219

[140] Sheu J, Hsiao G, Shen M, Fong T, Chen Y. Mechanisms involved in the antiplatelet activity of magnesium in human platelets. British Journal of Haematology. 2002;**119**:1033-1041

[141] Gawaz M, Ott I, Reininger AJ, Neumann FJ. Effects of magnesium on platelet aggregation and adhesion. Thrombosis and Haemostasis. 1994;**72**(6):912-918

[142] Ravn HB, Kristensen SD, Vissinger H, Husted SE. Magnesium Inhibits Human Platelets. Blood Coagulation & Fibrinolysis. 1996;**7**:241-244

[143] Hwang DL, Yen CF, Nadler JL. Effect of extracellular magnesium on platelet activation and intracellular calcium mobilization. American Journal of Hypertension. 1992;**5**:700-706

[144] Van Dijk PR, Waanders F, Qiu J, De Boer HHR, Van Goor H, Bilo HJG. Hypomagnesemia in persons with type 1 diabetes : Associations with clinical parameters and oxidative stress. Therapeutic Advances in Endocrinology and Metabolism. 2020;**11**:1-9. DOI: 10.1177/https

[145] Violi F, Pignatelli P, Basili S. Nutrition , supplements , and vitamins in platelet function and bleeding. Circulation. 2010;**121**:1033-1044. DOI: 10.1161/CIRCULATIONAHA.109.880211

[146] Homoncik M, Blann AD, Hollenstein U, Pernerstorfer T. Systemic inflammation increases shear stress-induced platelet plug formation measured by the PFA-100. British Journal of Haematology. 2000;**111**:1250-1252

[147] Poulsen TS, Mickley H. Is the antiplatelet effect of aspirin affected by systemic inflammation? Annals of Hematology. 2004;**83**(11):728. DOI: 10.1007/s00277-004-0940-1

[148] Dash P, Singh VK, Gautam D, Pathak A, Kumar A. Aspirin resistance and blood biomarkers in predicting

ischemic stroke recurrence : An exploratory study. Brain Circulation. 2022;**8**:31-37. DOI: 10.4103/bc.bc

[149] Gragnano F, Sperlongano S, Golia E, Natale F, Bianchi R, Crisci M, et al. The role of von Willebrand factor in vascular inflammation: From pathogenesis to targeted therapy. Mediators of Inflammation. 2017;**2017**:5620314. DOI: 10.1155/2017/5620314. Epub 2017 May 28. PMID: 28634421; PMCID: PMC5467347

[150] Van Den Dries LWJ, Gruters RA, Van Der Borden SBCH. von Willebrand factor is elevated in HIV patients with a history of thrombosis. Frontiers in Microbiology. 2015;**6**(March):180. DOI: 10.3389/fmicb.2015.00180

[151] Graham SM et al. Elevated plasma von Willebrand factor levels are associated with subsequent ischemic stroke in persons with treated HIV infection. Open Forum Infectious Diseases. 2021;**1**:1-9. DOI: 10.1093/ofid/ofab521

[152] Denorme F, Vanhoorelbeke K, De Meyer SF. von Willebrand factor and platelet glycoprotein Ib : A Thromboinflammatory Axis in stroke. Frontiers in Immunology. 2019;**10**(December):2884. DOI: 10.3389/fimmu.2019.02884

[153] Estevez B, Du X. New concepts and mechanisms of platelet activation signaling. Physiology. 2017;**32**(2):162-177. DOI: 10.1152/physiol.00020.2016

[154] Bergmeier W, Stefanini L. Platelet ITAM signaling. Current Opinion in Hematology. 2013;**20**(5):445-450. DOI: 10.1097/MOH.0b013e3283642267

[155] Garibaldi BT et al. The immature platelet fraction in HIV patients with thrombocytopenia. Blood. 2007;**110**(11):2095-2095. DOI: 10.1182/blood.v110.11.2095.2095

[156] Vaughan JL. Reticulated Platelet Fraction Levels in HIV Infected Individuals with Thrombocytopenia. Johanesburg: Witswatersrand; 2010

[157] Hamad MA, Schanze N, Schommer N, Nührenberg T, Duerschmied D. Reticulated platelets—Which functions have been established by in vivo and in vitro data? Cell. 2021;**10**(5):1172. DOI: 10.3390/cells10051172

[158] Rocca B et al. Modulation of the expression and activity of cyclooxygenases in normal and accelerated erythropoiesis. Experimental Hematology. 2004;**32**(10):925-934. DOI: 10.1016/j.exphem.2004.07.010

[159] Hsue PY. Mechanisms of cardiovascular disease in the setting of HIV infection. The Canadian Journal of Cardiology. 2019;**35**(3):238-248. DOI: 10.1016/j.cjca.2018.12.024

[160] Haissman JM, Haugaard AK, Ostrowski SR, Berge RK, Hov JR, Trøseid M, et al. Microbiota-dependent metabolite and cardiovascular disease marker trimethylamine-N-oxide (TMAO) is associated with monocyte activation but not platelet function in untreated HIV infection. BMC Infectious Diseases. 2017;**17**(1):445. DOI: 10.1186/s12879-017-2547-x

[161] Zhang X, Zhang X, Tong F, Cai Y, Zhang Y, Song H, et al. Gut microbiota induces high platelet response in patients with ST segment elevation myocardial infarction after ticagrelor treatment. eLife. 2022;**11**:e70240. DOI: 10.7554/eLife.70240

[162] Mak KH et al. Ethnic variation in adverse cardiovascular outcomes

and bleeding complications in the Clopidogrel for high Atherothrombotic risk and ischemic stabilization, management, and avoidance (CHARISMA) study. American Heart Journal. 2009;**157**(4):658-665. DOI: 10.1016/j.ahj.2008.08.031

[163] Goodman T, Ferro A, Sharma P. Pharmacogenetics of aspirin resistance: A comprehensive systematic review. British Journal of Clinical Pharmacology. 2008;**66**(2):222-232. DOI: 10.1111/j.1365-2125.2008.03183.x

[164] Pendyala LK et al. Racial disparity with on-treatment platelet reactivity in patients undergoing percutaneous coronary intervention. American Heart Journal. 2013;**166**(2):266-272. DOI: 10.1016/j.ahj.2013.04.008

[165] Infeld M et al. Platelet reactivity in response to aspirin and ticagrelor in African-Americans and European-Americans. Journal of Thrombosis and Thrombolysis. 2021;**51**(2):249-259. DOI: 10.1007/s11239-020-02327-w

[166] Nguyen TA, Diodati JG, Pharand C. Resistance to clopidogrel: A review of the evidence. Journal of the American College of Cardiology. 2005;**45**(8):1157-1164. DOI: 10.1016/j.jacc.2005.01.034

[167] Bazargan M, Wisseh C, Adinkrah E, Boyce S, King EO, Assari S. Low-dose aspirin use among African American older adults. Journal of American Board of Family Medicine. 2021;**34**(1):132-143. DOI: 10.3122/jabfm.2021.01.200322

[168] Bigna JJ, Noubiap JJ. The rising burden of non-communicable diseases in sub-Saharan Africa. Lancet Global Health. 2019;**7**(10):e1295-e1296. DOI: 10.1016/S2214-109X(19)30370-5

[169] Patel P et al. Noncommunicable diseases among HIV-infected persons in low-income and middle-income countries: A systematic review and meta-analysis. AIDS. 2018;**32**(November 2017):S5-S20. DOI: 10.1097/QAD.0000000000001888

[170] Mallick S, Shroff GR, Linzer M. Aspirin for primary prevention of cardiovascular disease: What do the current USPSTF guidelines say? Cleveland Clinic Journal of Medicine. 2023;**90**(5):287-291. DOI: 10.3949/ccjm.90a.22087

[171] Martinez E. Time to change cardiovascular prevention in people with HIV. Lancet HIV. 2019;**6**(12):e811-e812. DOI: 10.1016/S2352-3018(19)30329-7

[172] Jacobson MC, Dezube BJ, Aboulafia DM. Thrombotic complications in patients infected with HIV in the era of highly active antiretroviral therapy: A case series. Clinical Infectious Diseases. 2004;**39**(8):1214-1222. DOI: 10.1086/424664

[173] Burkholder GA et al. Underutilization of aspirin for primary prevention of cardiovascular disease among HIV-infected patients. Clinical Infectious Diseases. 2012;**55**(11):1550-1557. DOI: 10.1093/cid/cis752

[174] Suchindran S, Regan S, Meigs JB, Grinspoon SK, Triant VA. Aspirin use for primary and secondary prevention in human Immunode fi ciency virus (HIV)—Infected and HIV-uninfected patients. Open Forum Infectious Diseases. 2014;**1**(3):ofu076-ofu076. DOI: 10.1093/ofid/ofu076

[175] De Socio GV, Ricci E, Parruti G, Calza L, Maggi P, Celesia BM, et al. Statins and aspirin use in HIV-infected people: Gap between European AIDS clinical society guidelines and clinical practice: The results from HIV-HY

study. Infection. 2016;**44**(5):589-597. DOI: 10.1007/s15010-016-0893-z

[176] Maggi P et al. Use of statins and aspirin to prevent cardiovascular disease among HIV-positive patients. A survey among Italian HIV physicians. The New Microbiologica. 2017;**40**(2):139-142

[177] Ladapo JA, Richards AK, DeWitt CM, Harawa NT, Shoptaw S, Cunningham WE, et al. Disparities in the quality of cardiovascular care between HIV-infected versus HIV-uninfected adults in the United States: A cross-sectional study. Journal of the American Heart Association. 2017;**6**(11):e007107. DOI: 10.1161/JAHA.117.007107

[178] Cofer LB, Barrett TJ, Berger JS. Aspirin for the primary prevention of cardiovascular disease: Time for a platelet-guided approach. Arteriosclerosis, Thrombosis, and Vascular Biology. 2022;**42**(10):1207-1216. DOI: 10.1161/ATVBAHA.122.318020

[179] Berger JS. Aspirin for primary prevention—Time to rethink our approach. JAMA Network Open. 2022;**5**(Cvd):E2210144. DOI: 10.1001/jamanetworkopen.2022.10144

Chapter 3

Gene Therapy Approaches in HIV Treatment

Sachin Kothawade, Vaibhav Wagh, Vishal Pande and Amit Lunkad

Abstract

The search for a cure for human immunodeficiency virus (HIV) infection has been a persistent challenge in global health. While antiretroviral therapy (ART) has significantly improved the prognosis for individuals living with HIV, the need for lifelong treatment and the presence of viral reservoirs and drug resistance necessitate innovative approaches. Gene therapy has emerged as a promising avenue in HIV treatment, utilizing genetic modification to address the complexities of the virus. This chapter provides a comprehensive overview of gene therapy approaches in HIV treatment. It explores the fundamental principles and techniques of gene therapy and highlights the specific challenges posed by HIV. Various gene therapy strategies, including gene editing technologies and gene transfer methods, are discussed in detail, along with their potential advantages and limitations. Safety, efficacy, and ethical considerations in gene therapy for HIV are also examined. The chapter concludes with a glimpse into the future of gene therapy in HIV treatment, emphasizing the importance of interdisciplinary collaboration and continued research. This chapter aims to inspire further exploration and harnessing of gene therapy's transformative potential in the quest for an HIV cure.

Keywords: gene therapy, HIV, antiretroviral therapy, CRISPR/Cas9, viral reservoirs, gene editing

1. Introduction

Products for cell and gene therapy have been created and studied as possible therapies or cures for the HIV illness during the course of more than 20 years of study [1]. Here, we review recent developments and show how cell and gene therapies may be able to provide the coveted treatment.

HIV cell and gene therapy dates at least as far back as 1994, when a retroviral vector to rewire T cells such that they would express an MHC-unrestricted recognition protein [2]. The modified cells were designed to recognize and eliminate cells with infection that expressed cell surface envelope glycoprotein. The recognition molecule was a shortened variant of the CD4 glycoprotein receptor for (human immunodeficiency virus) HIV. This was an early version of what is now known as MHC-unrestricted and CAR-mediated recognition of cellular antigens. In the years that followed, T cells were modified to recognize infected cells via a variety of receptors, to fend against HIV attachment, and to prevent viral reproduction. Circulating lymphocytes or hematopoietic stem cell precursor cells (HSCPC) have undergone genetic changes, and cells were infused during clinical trials to see whether they might prevent the comeback of plasma viremia after treatment discontinuation [3]. Stable suppression of HIV in the absence of antiretroviral medication treatment has not been accomplished, with the exception of cells altered ex vivo to disrupt the CCR5 gene and infused into a trial participant heterozygous for the CCR5delta32 loss of function allele [4–6].

We provide this important evaluation of the most recent advances in gene and cell therapy for HIV to explain why so many approaches have failed to achieve the aim and if novel therapies have better chances. Studies on bulk CD4 T cell genetic manipulation, mostly employing CRISPR/Cas9 editing tools, and recent advancements in CAR methods, which are addressed elsewhere in this book, were purposefully left out [7–9].

Traditionally, there are two categories of gene therapy: those in which the effector molecule is a nucleic acid and those in which it is a protein. Based on how genetic treatment works, there is a second categorization. Thus, there are immunomodulatory proteins, suicide genes, ribozymes, decoy RNAs, DNA and RNA-based antisense compounds, and transdominant negative proteins.

1.1 Nucleic acid-based antivirals

1.1.1 Antisense

A definition of intracellular immunization as being more similar to traditional medications does not suit DNA oligonucleotides well. However, the idea of a particular treatment binding to a viral nucleic acid becomes highly alluring when you consider that a nucleotide sequence needs to be 17 bases to be unique within the human genome. Conventional DNA is fragile and challenging to work with. As a result, DNA oligonucleotides are often chemically altered bases with nuclease-resistant connections like phosphoroamidate or phosphorothioate. Tissue and cell penetration seems to be these compounds' main concern. An oligonucleotide's concentration is likely to decrease at least 10-fold from the extracellular to the intracellular compartment, and it loses even more concentration from the cytoplasm to the nucleus, where it has the greatest potential to have a therapeutic effect. Levin and Stein talk about these issues. Commercial businesses are still conducting clinical studies using GEM®91, a 25 nucleotide phosphorothioate oligodeoxynucleotide targeted at the gag start codon [10].

1.1.2 RNA based antivirals

1.1.2.1 Antisense RNA

This complementary RNA binds by Watson-Crick bands to the target RNA, generating a double-stranded structure that will be broken down by cellular enzymes. Naturally, areas of the HIV genome known to have significant cis-acting (non-coding) activities are the focus of antisense RNA strategies [11, 12]. As a result, popular targets include the TAR region/polyadenylation signal and the packaging signal. It has also been tried to use RNA directed against the coding sequences of several structural proteins and essential viral proteins including Tat and Rev. as depicted in **Figure 1** [13].

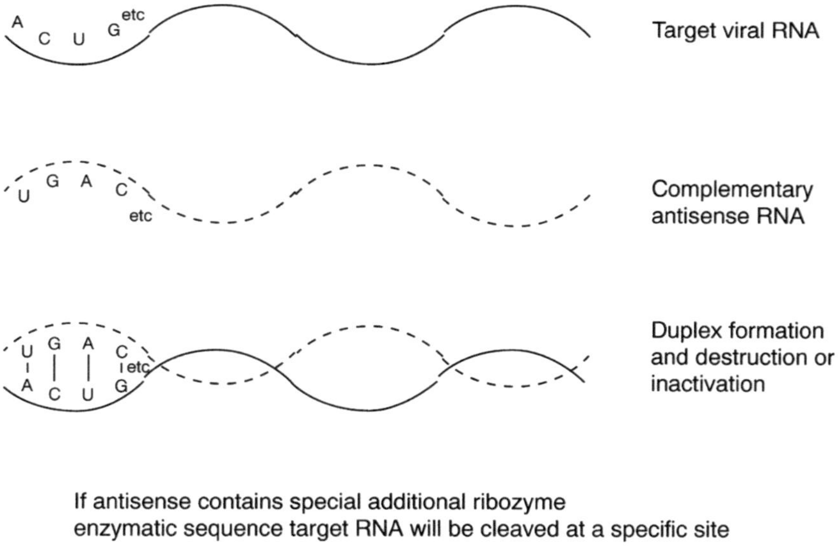

Figure 1.
Antisense and ribozymes.

Inhibiting HIV replication utilizing a range of delivery methods, such as microinjection or cotransfection of the antiviral with a DNA encoding the viral genes, has been shown in the majority of these investigations. Resistance to an HIV challenge has also been tested using cells that persistently produce antiviral antisense. The findings show some inconsistencies. For instance, targeting the RNA sequence responsive to Tat (TAR) and inhibiting the Tat initiation codon are thought to have a comparable impact [14]. This is not the case, which stresses how difficult it is to forecast how these molecules will interact with biological systems and how some of these agents' outcomes are not always reproducible.

1.1.2.2 Ribozyme antivirals

As with antisense, ribozymes bind to their target RNA by sequence complementarity, but they also include a unique sequence that functions like a typical enzyme and precisely cleaves the target RNA, making it inactive as depicted in **Figure 1**. These have mostly been reported to have comparable reported effectiveness and have been targeted against similar sections of the genome to those of antisense as well as the Rev. responsive element (RRE) [15]. As a catalytic agent, ribozymes are expected to have a stronger impact at lower concentrations since they may recycle and cleave subsequent target RNAs. This has not always been the case, and it is well known that ribozyme activity validated in vitro does not always correspond to effective function in cells. This is because some of the effect observed may be caused by an antisense effect of the complementary regions of the target and effector RNAs. The significance of the effector RNA's co-localization with its target RNA inside the cell does seem to have been verified as a principle. This has been accomplished by comparing the effects of targeted and non-targeted ribozymes and demonstrating a substantial difference between them.

A Phase I clinical study is being conducted on a hairpin ribozyme that targets the U5 region of the long terminal repeat and has been examined in vitro and in a

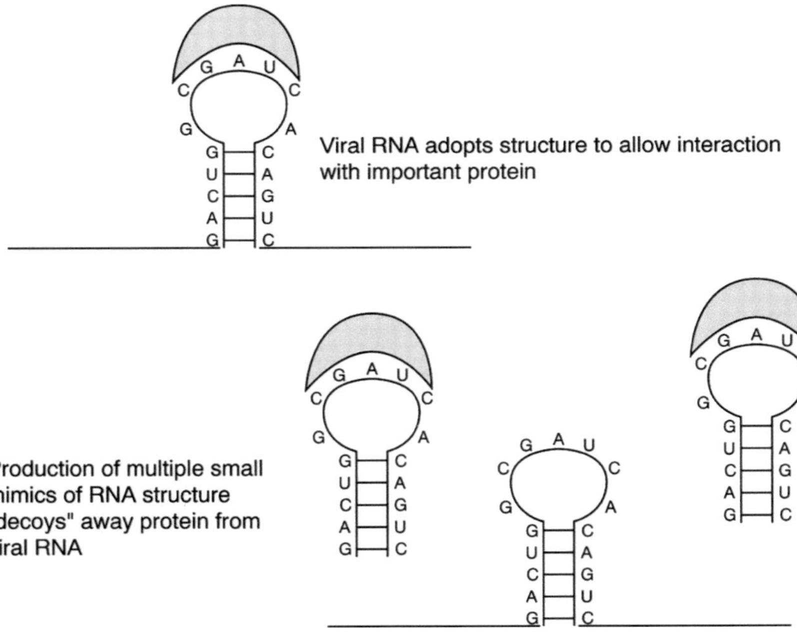

Figure 2.
Decoy strategy.

transgenic mouse model [16]. Additionally, some early findings indicate that an anti-Tat ribozyme-containing vector can increase the patient cells' ability to survive an HIV challenge.

1.1.2.3 Decoys

A crucial functional portion of the native viral RNA may adopt a structure similar to an RNA that can be expressed in a cell as a decoy (see **Figure 2**). The viral or cellular protein that is expected to interact with the viral RNA but is sequestered away by high levels of decoy expression, inhibiting proper viral processing. The TAR and the RRE have been apparent targets as could be predicted, and this method has shown some promising in vitro findings. Also investigated were decoys with the exact same structure as the packing signal (Ψ). Inhibiting viral replication is not consistently shown to be beneficial across all trials, however [17].

1.1.3 Protein based therapies

1.1.3.1 Transdominant proteins

A transdominant protein is a comparable but altered variant of the wild type protein that disrupts a viral process. Examples of this include structural proteins that help assemble multimeric complexes yet hinder the binding of additional subunits by their inclusion (see **Figure 3**). Alternately, a protein with a binding and an activation domain in its natural form may have the latter altered such that it will still bind but prevents the target from binding the original protein, preventing the necessary

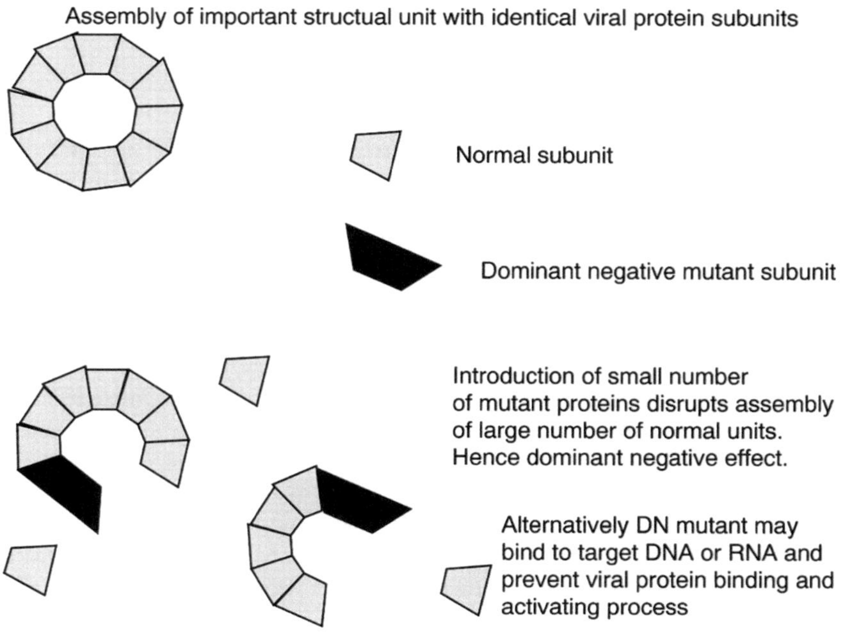

Figure 3.
Dominant negative inhibition.

process from occurring [18]. Transdominant inhibition is the term used to describe situations where a small number of units may counteract the effects of many wild type molecules. The Rev. M10 dominant mutant, which has been found to suppress laboratory and clinical viral isolates, is the one that has been examined the most in relation to HIV [19]. Since the M10 mutation affects Rev's nuclear export signal, it is likely interfering with its capacity to transport RNA out of the nucleus. Phase II clinical trials for Rev. M10 have begun, and preliminary findings from experiments reveal that cells expressing Rev. M10 outlive those expressing an inactive M10 version in vivo. A very little improvement has been made in the cellular half-life, which has been increased to a maximum of 15 days. In a similar vein, Sam, a mutant variant of Rev's cellular homolog, has been altered to join Rev. in an inactive complex. The possibility of interfering with vital physiological processes is one risk associated with the mutation of cellular proteins.

1.1.3.2 Transcellular antibodies

When attaching to their molecular targets, antibodies are very selective, and the production of a shortened version of the antibody—which will stay within the cell—has been utilized to target viral proteins and stop viral export. Working with antibodies against the viral envelope and reverse transcriptase enzyme, an anti-Tat antibody has been investigated. Similarly, a possible strategy utilizing this mechanism is to downregulate cell surface receptors like CXCR4 to obstruct viral entrance [20]. Again, however, suppressing the expression of a receptor that is vital for cell survival or performs important signaling activities might be dangerous.

1.1.3.3 Death genes

Incorporating a promoter that will be activated by the viral transactivator Tat (also known as the viral LTR) and drive a gene, such as a toxin or the thymidine kinase gene, which is fatal to cells in the presence of the medication ganciclovir, is an appealing alternative [21]. Although in principle this makes sense, the viral long terminal repeat has a very low level of specificity and is susceptible to activation by a variety of different viral and cellular transactivators. This will probably result in the somewhat non-specific killing of antiviral-expressing cells up until fine specificity of expression is attained.

1.1.3.4 Interferons

Natural antiviral chemicals called interferons are created in response to viral infection and other stimuli. The prospect of inhibiting viral replication by integrating the interferon gene under the control of the HIV-1 promoter or by utilizing the same promoter to drive interferon triggered antiviral enzymes like PKR has been investigated in a number of research [22]. Continuous low dosage interferon expression has also been studied and is thought to have a role in the broad and potent inhibition of viral replication. It seemed to have no negative effects on the transplanted human immune system cells in a mouse model [23].

2. Gene editing tools for HIV treatment

2.1 Introduction to gene editing technologies

Researchers now have the capacity to quickly and affordably incorporate sequence-specific alterations into the genomes of a variety of cell types and species because to the development of highly adaptable genome-editing methods. Transcription activator-like effector nucleases (TALENs), zinc-finger nucleases (ZFNs), clustered regularly interspaced short palindromic repeats (CRISPR)-CRISPR-associated protein 9 (Cas9), and homing endonucleases or meganucleases round out the core technologies that are currently most frequently used to facilitate genome editing (**Figure 4**) [24, 25].

2.2 CRISPR-Cas9 and its applications in targeting the viral genome

CRISPR stands for clustered regularly interspaced short palindromic repeats, which were discovered to be separated by spacers—non-repeating DNA sequences—in *Escherichia coli*. The memory of the plasmid and phage genomes is provided by these spacers, known as CRISPR arrays, which were subsequently identified as acquired copies of previously encountered foreign DNA. The bacteria create RNA segments from the CRISPR arrays to target the pathogen specifically and launch an adaptive immune response when they come into contact with the foreign genetic material once again. Well-conserved CRISPR-associated (Cas) genes around CRISPR arrays have been classified into families and subtypes based on the closeness of their encoded proteins' sequences. There are six different CRISPR/Cas system varieties, which have been split into two groups: in class two systems (types II, V, and VI), interference is carried out by a single effector protein as opposed to class 1 systems (types I, III, and IV), which use multi-Cas protein complexes [26, 27].

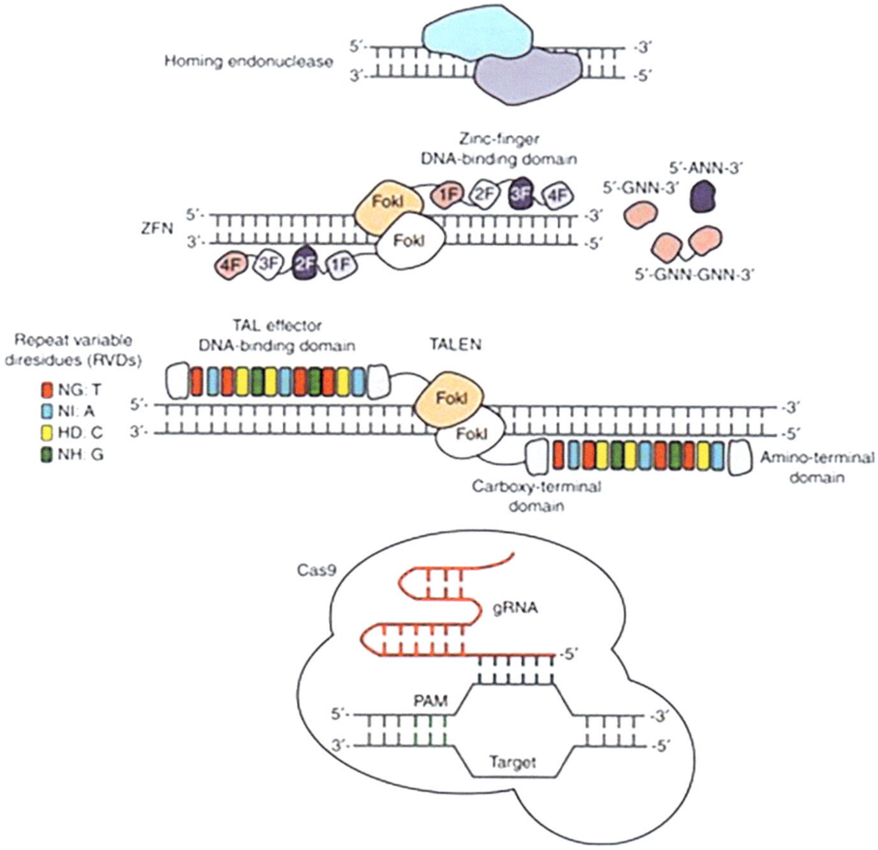

Figure 4.
Genome-editing technologies.

The Streptococcus pyogenes (Sp) Type II CRISPR/Cas9 system is the one that has been investigated and utilized the most. The CRISPR/Cas9 system's overall biogenesis and operation are shown in **Figure 5**. The unique protospacer sequences found in the CRISPR array, which have similarity to foreign DNA, are translated to create lengthy precursor CRISPR RNA (pre-crRNA). The interference apparatus is subsequently directed by the pre-crRNA to cleave complementary sequences or protospacers, thus eradicating the foreign DNA. In order to bind crRNA in a sequence complementary way and draw in the RNAse III and CRISPR-associated nine (Cas9) enzymes, an invariant trans-activating CRISPR RNA (tracrRNA) is needed [28]. TracrRNA, RNAse III, and Cas9 combine to create a complex with every distinct crRNA. This system's protospacer adjacent motifs (PAMs), which are situated just where the crRNA would bind, are essential and help to make CRISPR targeting specific. Invading foreign DNA is removed by genome editing processes involving non-homologous end joining (NHEJ) or homology-directed repair (HDR), which are stimulated by the helicase and nuclease activity of Cas protein motifs that are guided by crRNA [29].

The Cas9 effector endonuclease has been repurposed by scientists as a pharmaceutical tool for accurate gene editing to remove or integrate specific genes in the human genome. The tracrRNA:crRNA complex has been amalgamated into a single guide RNA (sgRNA) to direct CRISPR-Cas9 toward the intended genomic targets [30].

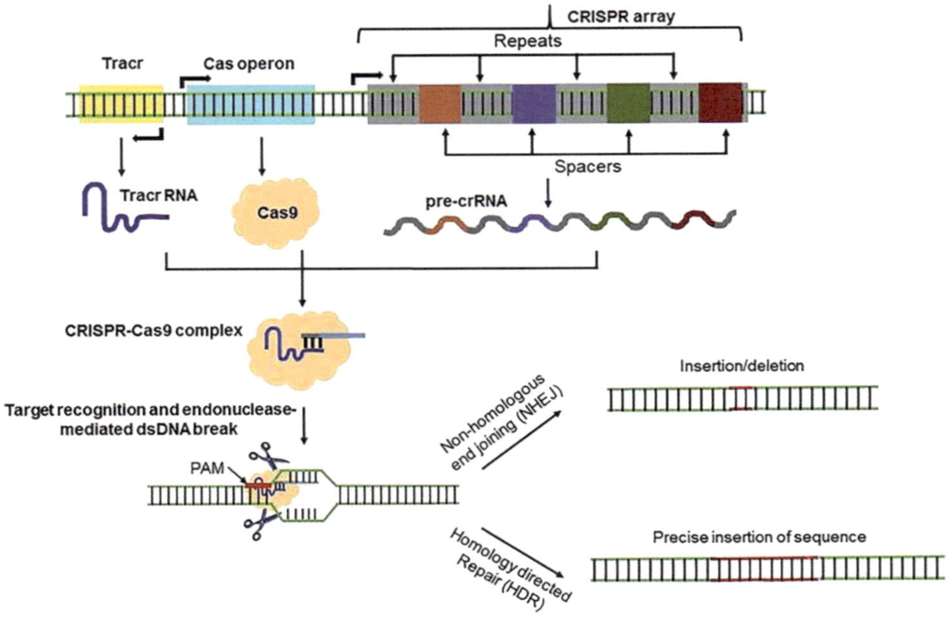

Figure 5.
Outline of guiding RNA biosynthesis and CRISPR-Cas9 genome targeting. The essential elements of Streptococcus pyogenes site for CRISPR-Cas.

The successful utilization of this system and its gene editing capabilities in eukaryotic cells has led to its widespread adoption in various research domains. CRISPR/Cas9 is now a commonly employed technique.

3. In vivo gene therapy strategies

Using in vivo gene transfer techniques, the gene therapy vector is either administered directly to the target organ or is delivered via the vascular system to the organ's feeding channels. Compared to ex vivo methods, in vivo gene transfer offers the benefit of avoiding the time-consuming (and expensive) procedure of extracting cells from the patient, genetically altering the cells in vitro, and then returning the transformed cells to the patient. The induction of immunity by the gene transfer vector, delivery of the gene therapy vector to the targeted cells/organs, effective binding of the vector to the cell, translocation of the genetic material to the nucleus, and toxicity and immunity induced by virus expression are obstacles that need to be overcome for in vivo gene transfer strategies as depicted in **Figure 6** [31].

3.1 Delivery methods for in vivo gene therapy

Different techniques are used by gene delivery systems to enable the absorption of the gene that has been chosen to target the cell. A thorough knowledge of the interaction process between the target cell and the delivery system is necessary for the effective design of a gene delivery system. The key to creating a more efficient gene delivery system is comprehending intercellular flow and targeting mechanisms.

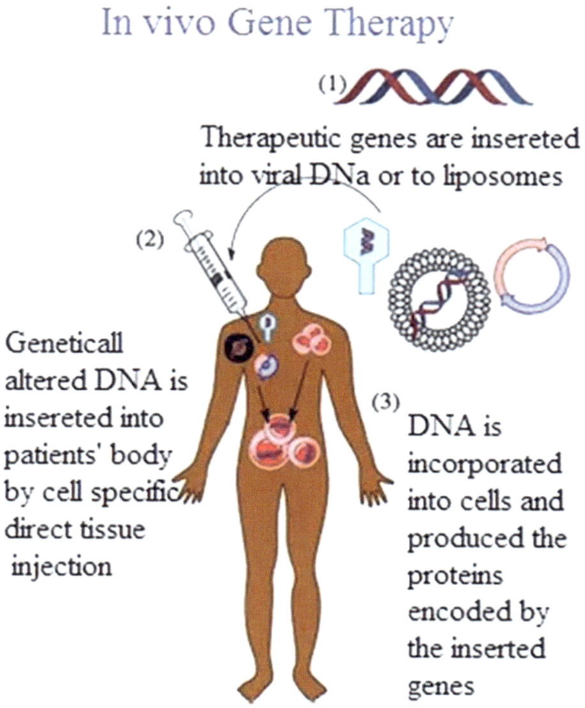

Figure 6.
In vivo gene therapy.

Cell targeting is the process of delivering a therapeutic substance to a particular cell organelle or compartment. In endocytosis gene therapy, especially in cellular absorption of non-viral gene delivery methods, it is the most often employed technique. Viral gene delivery systems are made up of viruses that have undergone engineering to become replication-deficient. These viruses are able to carry the genes to the cells for expression. For the delivery of viral genes, lentiviruses, retroviruses, and adenoviruses are used. The continual expression and expression of therapeutic genes are benefits of viral systems. The utilization of these systems is however constrained by certain drawbacks, including the creation of viruses, immunogenicity, toxicity, and lack of optimization in large-scale manufacturing [32–34].

As an alternative to systems based on viruses, non-viral gene delivery methods were created. These systems' ability to develop transfection is one of their key benefits. Physical and chemical delivery methods for non-viral genes are separated into these two groups. The most popular physical techniques include microinjection, electroporation, gene guns, ultrasound-mediated techniques, and hydrodynamic systems. Physical techniques entail applying physical pressure to make the cell membrane more permeable so that the gene may enter the cell. Physical approaches' main benefits are that they are dependable and simple to utilize. They can also injure tissue in particular situations, which is a drawback.

For gene transport into the cell, chemical approaches employ carriers made from synthetic or natural chemicals, such as synthetic and natural polymers, liposomes, dendrimers, synthetic proteins, and cationic lipids. The fact that these systems are non-immunogenic and often have minimal toxicity is one of their main benefits [35].

In vivo gene therapy	Ex vivo gene therapy
Another type of gene therapy is in vivo gene therapy, which is done directly when the defective cells are yet in the body.	Ex vivo gene therapy is a type of gene therapy in which gene modification is done outside the patient's body.
It is less invasive	It is more invasive
Technically simple	Technically more complex
Vectors introduced directly in body	No vectors introduced directly in body
In this method safety check is not possible	In this method safety check is possible
Decreased control over target cells	Close control possible

Table 1.
Difference between in vivo and ex vivo gene therapy.

The difference between in vivo and ex vivo gene therapy as given in **Table 1**.

3.2 Viral vectors and their role in delivering therapeutic genes

According to whether their genomes integrate into the host cellular chromatin (oncoretroviruses and Lentivirus) or remain in the cell nucleus mostly as extra chromosomal episomes (Adeno-Associated Virus, Adenovirus, and herpes viruses), the five main classes of viral vectors may be divided into two categories. The effectiveness of transgenic expression, simplicity of manufacture, safety, toxicity, and stability all factor into the selection of viral vectors for clinical usage.

Additionally, RNA and DNA viruses with either single-stranded (ss) or double-stranded (ds) genomes serve as examples of the various vector types. Eight Infectious agents are categorized into risk groups for laboratory research (Risk Groups 1–4) in the World Health Organization (WHO) Laboratory Biosafety Manual and the National Institutes of Health (NIH) Recombinant DNA Guidelines. The risk group provides information on the biosafety degree of containment required to reduce risk while handling certain infectious pathogens.

3.2.1 Adenovirus vector

Adenoviruses are a group of non-enveloped DNA viruses with double-stranded genomes that range in size from 34 to 43 kb. These viruses use alternative splicing to encode genes in both sense and antisense directions. The AV genome has eight transcription units and two ITRs on either side of it. The first viral sections to be transcriptionally transcribed are known as the early regions (E1A, E1B, E2, E3, and E4), which also include the proteins that activate transcription of additional viral regions and modify the cellular environment to enhance viral production [36]. From an alternatively spliced transcript, the late sections (L1-L5) are translated. After infection, the AV genome persists in an additional chromosomal form. Humans have 51 different serotypes of AV; 45–80% of the population harbors neutralizing antibodies against Ad5, the most prevalent, due to natural infections, which typically date back to infancy [37]. They are capable of high titer production and high infection multiplicity gene delivery. These characteristics have made them one of the viral vectors most often utilized in in vivo research and clinical trials for gene therapy. Adenoviral vectors can, however, cause a large amount of inflammation, which severely restricts their practical application. Additionally, because adenoviral vectors cannot integrate into the host's genome, the transgene's expression is episomal and hence transitory. Due to this drawback, adenoviral vectors are more frequently utilized to create short-term gene expression than they are for illnesses that call for continuous gene expression. Adenoviral vectors, for instance, are used in cancer research to transmit a suicide gene that kills tumor cells [38].

3.2.2 Retrovirus vector

Retroviruses have a diploid ssRNA genome, an enveloped RNA structure, and at least 4 genes: gag, pro, pol, and env. The major structural polyprotein, which is encoded by the gag gene, is required for the formation of immature and non-infectious viral-like particles [39]. The viral protease, which is encoded by the pro gene, aids in the development of viral particles. Reverse transcriptase, RNase H, and integrase are made by the pol gene, whereas the env gene makes the viral surface glycoproteins and transmembrane proteins that facilitate binding to cellular receptors and membrane fusion. The capacity of RV and retroviral vectors to incorporate into host DNA is a common characteristic. In addition, complex RV like HIV-1 encode auxiliary proteins that improve replication and contagiousness. Reversible transcription of viral RNA results in integration of the transcript into a provirus. The host cell's enzymes are extremely successfully used by the RV for both long-term production of viral proteins and replication. Like the majority of viruses, the RV requires a receptor to enter the host cell. Many oncogenic RVs are replication-defective variants that include oncogene sequence in place of a portion of their normal viral gene complement. Malignant illness and a number of other pathogenic states are also brought on by replication-competent retroviruses in a wide range of animals. The acquired immunodeficiency syndrome (AIDS) is caused by the retrovirus's HIV-1 and HIV-2 [40].

Retroviruses display a number of properties/characteristics that influences their potential asvectors in gene therapy protocols. These may be summarized as follows:

- The biochemistry and molecular biology of retroviruses as a whole have been extensively investigated.
- The majority of retroviruses can only incorporate their proviral DNA into cells that are actively reproducing.
- The efficacy of gene transfer to the most vulnerable cell types is extremely high, frequently close to 100%.
- It is possible for integrated DNA to experience persistent, somewhat high-level expression.
- The chromosomes of the host are randomly incorporated with proviral DNA.
- Retroviruses are promiscuous in that they infect a wide range of cell types that are dividing.
- If the original recipient cell splits, full copies of the proviral DNA are passed on to daughter cells.

- It is possible to create reliable, high-level titer stocks of replication-incompetent retroviral particles.
- Retroviral vectors have previously been the subject of several animal species' safety investigations.

The use of retroviruses as gene therapy vectors is nonetheless restricted by several of the other traits described. Their capacity to infect only dividing cells obviously limits their usage in the majority of cases.

Another drawback is that they are not selective about the kinds of proliferating cells that they infect. The entrance of each particular retrovirus is contingent upon the presence of an adequate viral receptor on the surface of a target cell, and they will not infect all types of proliferating cells. It is still challenging to forecast the full spectrum of cell types that any retrovirus is likely to infect during a gene therapy regimen since the identities of the majority of retroviral receptors are yet unknown. Physiological issues might arise if the foreign gene is integrated and expressed in cells other than the target cells as depicted in **Figure** 7.

In the context of gene therapy, clinical applications for monogenic disorders, cancer, and infectious illnesses, retroviral vectors have been widely utilized to transport therapeutic genes, ensuring a stable and effective expression of the transgene in patients [41].

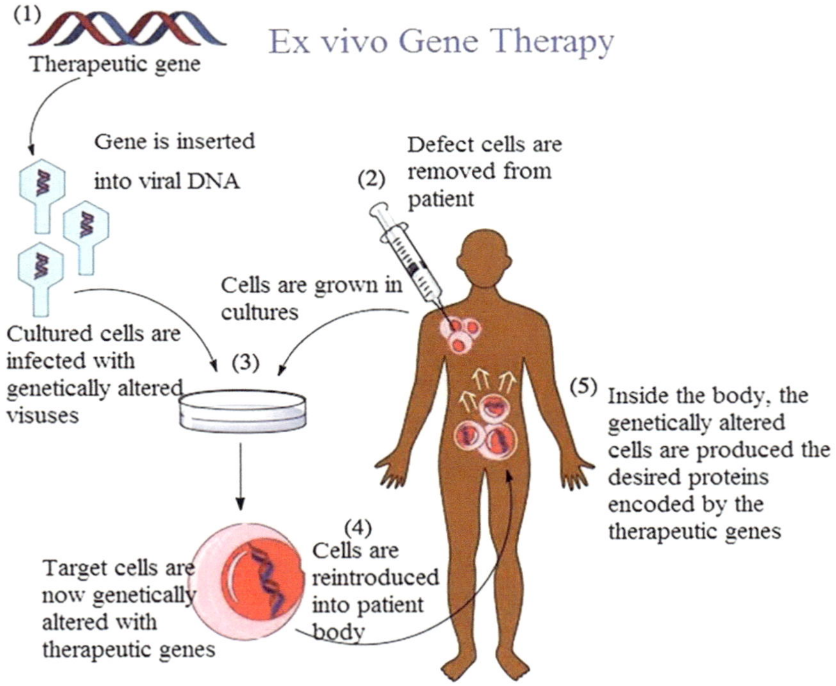

Figure 7.
Ex vivo gene therapy.

3.3 Modification of hematopoietic stem cells for enhanced antiviral properties

The treatment of an increasing variety of human illnesses with hematopoietic stem cell gene therapy (HSC GT) is proving to be an effective and adaptable method. After receiving a conditioning therapy that encourages their engraftment in the bone marrow, hematopoietic stem/progenitor cells (HSPC) are removed from the body, genetically modified ex vivo, and then reinjected back into the same person. The engrafted HSPC guarantee a consistent flow of genetically modified offspring, maybe throughout the recipient's whole life.

Then, mature cells from many lineages may treat diseases including cancer, infections, genetic immune weaknesses, and problems with blood and storage.

Treatment of numerous hematologic illnesses has shown effective when hematopoietic stem cells (HSCs) are genetically modified using lentiviral or anti-retroviral vectors (LVs). The degree of alteration of real repopulating HSCs continues to be a key determinant of therapy success. Gene delivery has been demonstrated to be improved by transduction-enhancing methods such as HSC-enhancing cytokine culture, high multiplicity of infection (MOI), repeated LV injection, alternative LV envelope pseudotyping, or the inclusion of transduction-enhancing small molecules [42].

Hematopoietic stem and progenitor cells (HSPCs) are resistant to infection by a variety of viruses and intracellular bacteria in addition to LV transduction. The significance of constitutive interferon-stimulated gene expression in pluripotent and multipotent cell types has recently come to light. The interferon-induced transmembrane (IFITM) family of proteins in particular, which are interferon-regulated innate effectors, offer an inherent defense against pathogens that depend on cellular endosomes for entrance and transport [43].

The IFITM proteins were initially discovered to be antiviral effectors against the vesicular stomatitis virus (VSV). They have the ability to limit the transduction of VSV-G protein pseudotyped (LV) LV and to control cellular growth, adhesion, and development. We recently shown that the mammalian target of rapamycin (mTOR) inhibitor rapamycin pharmacologically overcomes the IFITM limitation, which restricts the effectiveness of gene delivery using VSV-G pseudotyped LVs in HPSCs. Rapamycin, a substance that suppresses the immune system and has a variety of undesirable consequences, can cause cell growth to be delayed. Although they can have unfavorable cytotoxic effects, staurosporine and the IFITM3-modulating cyclosporines also exhibit LV transduction enhancer activity. The various restriction factors from HIV-1 trafficking that the VSV-G pseudotyped LVs experience as a result of their different subcellular trafficking approach might impact integration and change delay [44].

3.4 Genetic engineering of T cells for improved immune response

The gene transfer could be used to improve the effectiveness of T lymphocytes was apparent from the beginning of clinical studies in the field. T cells were the very first targets for genetic modification in human gene transfer experiments. An advantage of T cell-based immunotherapy compared to conventional chemotherapy, small molecules, and monoclonal antibodies is endurance because of continual generation of antigen-specific effector and memory T cells. In the presence of chronic infections or cancer, this hallmark allows both responses to pathogens and hiking for recurrence and minimal residual disease. However, persistence of genetically modified lymphocytes has been variable and often suboptimal in clinical trials. This variability may be a result of differences in the composition of infused cells, with some studies infusing a mixture of CD4+ and CD8+ cells, and other pure populations of CD8+ cytotoxic cells [45]. In addition, T cells may differ in their expansion potential, homing, and persistence, based on their differentiation status. When T lymphocytes encounter antigen, they undergo a developmental program from naïve (TNA), to central memory (TCM) and effector memory (TEM) cells. Gene-modified lymphocytes currently infused to patients are usually generated starting from unselected circulating T cells and will thus contain an unpredictable mixture of cellular subsets. Investigators are now trying to identify the optimal T cell target for gene transfer [46].

4. Safety and ethical considerations

The following elements should be considered in order to ensure the security of gene therapy for HIV: international cooperation between researchers from the public and private sectors, as well as participation from communities affected by the virus, social value, scientific validity, fair participant and study site selection, a favorable and acceptable risk-benefit balance, independent scientific and ethical review, informed and voluntary consent, and respect for enrolled patients. Participants should receive appropriate medical care and compensation if they suffer unpleasant study-related occurrences.

Genome editing technologies are regarded as the most challenging yet effective tools for gene therapy procedures [47]. Zinc finger nucleases (ZFN), transcription activator-like effector nucleases (TALEN), and clustered regularly interspaced short palindromic repeats (CRISPR)/CRISPR-associated protein 9 (Cas9) are the most widely used methods for editing the genome. The biggest moral problem with gene therapy is called "off-target mutation," which can lead to insertional mutagenesis and gene mutation. Because genome editing is a new and unpredictable technique and because the mechanisms regulating gene regulation and embryonic development are still poorly understood, bioethicists and scientists fear that the effects of germline therapy could be fatal [48]. Despite having demonstrated its value in therapeutic somatic applications, CRISPR/Cas has not yet advanced to the point where it may be utilized to alter the human genome for clinical reproductive purposes. As a result, the apparent long-term effects cannot be ignored. Genome editing on human embryos carries a very high risk of causing pathological diseases and disabilities, which may have long-term consequences for both the patient and their offspring. Off-target cleavage activity in DNA sequences has been demonstrated to occasionally occur in the past, despite stringent constraints on Cas9 targeting specificity [49].

Since the first gene therapy death in a clinical trial was announced in September 1999, the informed decision to participate in a clinical study has become more and more contentious. It is encouraged that patients in gene therapy clinical trials receive in-depth information about the potential dangers and benefits of the therapy in order to provide them the knowledge to make an informed decision about whether or not to participate without being forced [50]. The National Human Genome Research Institute (NHGRI) highlighted the requirement and significance of informed permission in CRISPR somatic genome editing after interviewing individuals with sickle cell disease for a study [51]. Though gene therapies may one day treat a wide range of terminal illnesses, the perceived benefits of the technology should not overshadow the difficulties patients may face in comprehending long-term hazards. While somatic gene therapy complies with the requirement for informed consent, the regulation of germline embryo editing raises more difficult issues, such as whether or not a future generation's consent is required and, if so, who should provide that consent given that embryos are unable to give their consent for germline intervention [51]. Regarding the extent of parental authority over the embryo, there is ethical discussion about whether parents will be the only autonomous entity to make decisions for their unborn children or if this will be seen as displacing the interests of future generations who are unable to consent at the time of the decision [52].

5. Conclusions

Gene therapy approaches in HIV treatment hold immense promise in addressing the challenges associated with the management and potential cure of human immunodeficiency virus (HIV) infection. This chapter has provided a comprehensive overview of the principles, techniques, and potential applications of gene therapy in the context of HIV.

The exploration of various gene therapy strategies, including gene editing technologies such as CRISPR/Cas9 and gene transfer methods utilizing viral and non-viral vectors, has shed light on the potential advantages and limitations of each approach. These advancements have opened up new avenues for targeted intervention, modification of viral reservoirs, and enhancement of the immune response against HIV.

Critical considerations surrounding the safety, efficacy, and ethical implications of gene therapy have been addressed. It is crucial to conduct rigorous preclinical and clinical evaluations to ensure the safety of these approaches and to monitor long-term effects. Additionally, ethical discussions must accompany the development and implementation of gene therapies to ensure responsible and equitable use.

Looking ahead, the future of gene therapy in HIV treatment holds significant potential. Continued interdisciplinary collaboration between researchers, clinicians, and policymakers is essential to advance the field and translate scientific discoveries into practical applications. Ongoing research, clinical trials, and technological advancements will further refine gene therapy approaches and increase their efficacy and accessibility. While challenges remain, including the need for efficient delivery systems, cost-effectiveness, and scalability, the progress made in gene therapy for HIV treatment offers hope for a potential cure. By harnessing the transformative power of gene therapy and building upon the knowledge gained, researchers and practitioners can strive toward improved outcomes for individuals living with HIV.

Acknowledgements

The authors would like to express their sincere gratitude to the Management of RSM's N. N. Sattha College of Pharmacy, Ahmednagar, for providing the necessary resources and support for the completion of this work. We would also like to acknowledge the valuable contributions of our colleagues who provided insightful discussions and suggestions throughout the research process.

Conflict of interest

The authors declare no conflict of interest.

Author details

Sachin Kothawade[1*], Vaibhav Wagh[1], Vishal Pande[1] and Amit Lunkad[2]

1 RSM's N.N. Sattha College of Pharmacy, Ahmednagar, MH, India

2 SCSSS's Sitabai Thite College of Pharmacy, Shirur, MH, India

*Address all correspondence to: sachin.kothawade23@gmail.com

IntechOpen

References

[1] Ferrua F, Cicalese MP, Galimberti S, Giannelli S, Dionisio F, Barzaghi F, et al. Lentiviral haemopoietic stem/progenitor cell gene therapy for treatment of Wiskott-Aldrich syndrome: Interim results of a non-randomised, open-label, phase 1/2 clinical study. The Lancet Haematology. 2019;**6**(5):e239-e253. DOI: 10.1016/S2352-3026(19)30021-3

[2] Roybal KT, Lim WA. Synthetic immunology: Hacking immune cells to expand their therapeutic capabilities. Annual Review of Immunology. 2017;**35**:229-253. DOI: 10.1146/annurev-immunol-051116-052302

[3] Sano S, Sano T, Ishigami S, Ito T. Cardiac stem cell therapy: Does a newborn infant's heart have infinite potential for stem cell therapy? The Journal of Thoracic and Cardiovascular Surgery. 2022;**163**(1):242-247. DOI: 10.1016/j.jtcvs.2020.07.124

[4] Kiem HP, Jerome KR, Deeks SG, McCune JM. Hematopoietic-stem-cell-based gene therapy for HIV disease. Cell Stem Cell. 2012;**10**(2):137-147. DOI: 10.1016/j.stem.2011.12.015

[5] Bullen CK, Laird GM, Durand CM, Siliciano JD, Siliciano RF. New ex vivo approaches distinguish effective and ineffective single agents for reversing HIV-1 latency in vivo. Nature Medicine. 2014;**20**(4):425-429. DOI: 10.1038/nm.3489

[6] Deeks SG, Archin N, Cannon P, Collins S, Jones RB, de Jong MA, et al. Research priorities for an HIV cure: International AIDS society global scientific strategy 2021. Nature Medicine. 2021;**27**(12):2085-2098. DOI: 10.1038/s41591-021-01590-5

[7] Hamilton JR, Tsuchida CA, Nguyen DN, Shy BR, McGarrigle ER, Espinoza CR, et al. Targeted delivery of CRISPR-Cas9 and transgenes enables complex immune cell engineering. Cell Reports. 2021;**35**(9):109207. DOI: 10.1016/j.celrep.2021.109207

[8] Rupp LJ, Schumann K, Roybal KT, Gate RE, Ye CJ, Lim WA, et al. CRISPR/Cas9-mediated PD-1 disruption enhances anti-tumor efficacy of human chimeric antigen receptor T cells. Scientific Reports. 2017;**7**(1):1-10. DOI: 10.1038/s41598-017-00462-8

[9] Hultquist JF, Hiatt J, Schumann K, McGregor MJ, Roth TL, Haas P, et al. CRISPR-Cas9 genome engineering of primary CD4+ T cells for the interrogation of HIV-host factor interactions. Nature Protocols. 2019;**14**(1):1-27. DOI: 10.1038/s41596-018-0069-7

[10] Mansoor M, Melendez AJ. Advances in antisense oligonucleotide development for target identification, validation, and as novel therapeutics. Gene Regulation and Systems Biology. 2008;**2**:GRSB-S418. DOI: 10.4137/GRSB.S418

[11] Kornienko AE, Guenzl PM, Barlow DP, Pauler FM. Gene regulation by the act of long non-coding RNA transcription. BMC Biology. 2013;**11**:1-4. DOI: 10.1186/1741-7007-11-59

[12] Li R, Caico I, Xu Z, Iqbal MS, Romerio F. Epigenetic regulation of HIV-1 sense and antisense transcription in response to latency-reversing agents. Non-Coding RNA. 2023;**9**(1):5. DOI: 10.3390/ncrna9010005

[13] Hu S, Jing Y, Li T, Wang YG, Liu Z, Gao J, et al. Inferring Circadian Gene

Regulatory Relationships from Gene Expression Data with a Hybrid Frame Work. 05 January 2023 preprint (Version 1) available at Research Square. DOI: 10.21203/rs.3.rs-2401108/v1

[14] Lalonde MS, Lobritz MA, Ratcliff A, Chamanian M, Athanassiou Z, Tyagi M, et al. Inhibition of both HIV-1 reverse transcription and gene expression by a cyclic peptide that binds the tat-transactivating response element (TAR) RNA. PLoS Pathogens. 2011;7(5):e1002038. DOI: 10.1371/journal.ppat.1002038

[15] Tazi J, Bakkour N, Marchand V, Ayadi L, Aboufirassi A, Branlant C. Alternative splicing: Regulation of HIV-1 multiplication as a target for therapeutic action. The FEBS Journal. 2010;**277**(4):867-876. DOI: 10.1111/j.1742-4658.2009.07522.x

[16] Reyes-Darias JA, Sánchez-Luque FJ, Berzal-Herranz A. Inhibition of HIV-1 replication by RNA-based strategies. Current HIV Research. 2008;**6**(6):500-514. DOI: 10.2174/157016208786501454

[17] Verkhivker GM, Agajanian S, Oztas DY, Gupta G. Allosteric control of structural mimicry and mutational escape in the SARS-CoV-2 spike protein complexes with the ACE2 decoys and miniprotein inhibitors: A network-based approach for mutational profiling of binding and signaling. Journal of Chemical Information and Modeling. 2021;**61**(10):5172-5191. DOI: 10.1021/acs.jcim.1c00766

[18] van Loo G, Saelens X, Van Gurp M, MacFarlane M, Martin SJ, Vandenabeele P. The role of mitochondrial factors in apoptosis: A Russian roulette with more than one bullet. Cell Death & Differentiation. 2002;**9**(10):1031-1042. DOI: 10.1038/sj.cdd.4401088

[19] Rossi JJ, June CH, Kohn DB. Genetic therapies against HIV. Nature Biotechnology. 2007;**25**(12):1444-1454. DOI: 10.1038/nbt1367

[20] Anderson J, Banerjea A, Planelles V, Akkina R. Potent suppression of HIV type 1 infection by a short hairpin anti-CXCR4 siRNA. AIDS Research and Human Retroviruses. 2003;**19**(8):699-706. DOI: 10.1089/088922203322280928

[21] Saeb S, Van Assche J, Loustau T, Rohr O, Wallet C, Schwartz C. Suicide gene therapy in cancer and HIV-1 infection: An alternative to conventional treatments. Biochemical Pharmacology. 2022;**197**:114893. DOI: 10.1016/j.bcp.2021.114893

[22] Porritt RA, Hertzog PJ. Dynamic control of type I IFN signalling by an integrated network of negative regulators. Trends in immunology. 2015;**36**(3):150-160. DOI: 10.1016/j.it.2015.02.002

[23] McCauley SM, Kim K, Nowosielska A, Dauphin A, Yurkovetskiy L, Diehl WE, et al. Intron-containing RNA from the HIV-1 provirus activates type I interferon and inflammatory cytokines. Nature Communications. 2018;**9**(1):5305. DOI: 10.1038/s41467-018-07753-2

[24] Gaj T, Sirk SJ, Shui SL, Liu J. Genome-editing technologies: Principles and applications. Cold Spring Harbor perspectives in biology. 2016;**8**(12):a023754. DOI: 10.1101/cshperspect.a023754

[25] Gaj T, Gersbach CA, Barbas CF. ZFN, TALEN, and CRISPR/Cas-based methods for genome engineering. Trends in Biotechnology. 2013;**31**(7):397-405. DOI: 10.1016/j.tibtech.2013.04.004

[26] Makarova KS, Wolf YI, Iranzo J, Shmakov SA, Alkhnbashi OS, Brouns SJ, et al. Evolutionary classification of

CRISPR-Cas systems: A burst of class 2 and derived variants. Nature Reviews Microbiology. 2020;**18**(2):67-83. DOI: 10.1038/s41579-019-0299-x

[27] Chaudhuri A, Halder K, Datta A. Classification of CRISPR/Cas system and its application in tomato breeding. Theoretical and Applied Genetics. 2022;**135**(2):367-387. DOI: 10.1007/s00122-021-03984-y

[28] Moon SB, Kim DY, Ko JH, Kim YS. Recent advances in the CRISPR genome editing tool set. Experimental & Molecular Medicine. 2019;**51**(11):1-11. DOI: 10.1038/s12276-019-0339-7

[29] Shmakov S, Abudayyeh OO, Makarova KS, Wolf YI, Gootenberg JS, Semenova E, et al. Discovery and functional characterization of diverse class 2 CRISPR-Cas systems. Molecular Cell. 2015;**60**(3):385-397. DOI: 10.1016/j.molcel.2015.10.008

[30] Kaushik I, Ramachandran S, Srivastava SK. CRISPR-Cas9: A multifaceted therapeutic strategy for cancer treatment. In: Seminars in Cell & Developmental Biology. Vol. 96. Academic Press; 2019. pp. 4-12. DOI: 10.1016/j.semcdb.2019.04.018

[31] Mendell JR, Al-Zaidy SA, Rodino-Klapac LR, Goodspeed K, Gray SJ, Kay CN, et al. Current clinical applications of in vivo gene therapy with AAVs. Molecular Therapy. 2021;**29**(2):464-488. DOI: 10.1016/j.ymthe.2020.12.007

[32] Lee CS, Bishop ES, Zhang R, Yu X, Farina EM, Yan S, et al. Adenovirus-mediated gene delivery: Potential applications for gene and cell-based therapies in the new era of personalized medicine. Genes & diseases. 2017;**4**(2):43-63. DOI: 10.1016/j.gendis.2017.04.001

[33] Wang D, Tai PW, Gao G. Adeno-associated virus vector as a platform for gene therapy delivery. Nature Reviews Drug Discovery. 2019;**18**(5):358-378. DOI: 10.1038/s41573-019-0012-9

[34] Verma IM, Somia N. Gene therapy-promises, problems and prospects. Nature. 1997;**389**(6648):239-242. DOI: 10.1038/38410

[35] Cevher E, Demir A, Sefik E. Gene Delivery Systems: Recent Progress in Viral and Non-Viral Therapy [Internet]. Recent Advances in Novel Drug Carrier Systems. London, UK: InTech; 2012. DOI: 10.5772/53392

[36] Fonseca GJ, Cohen MJ, Mymryk JS. Adenovirus E1A recruits the human Paf1 complex to enhance transcriptional elongation. Journal of Virology. 2014;**88**(10):5630-5637. DOI: 10.1128/JVI.03518-13

[37] Rodrigues GA, Shalaev E, Karami TK, Cunningham J, Slater NK, Rivers HM. Pharmaceutical development of AAV-based gene therapy products for the eye. Pharmaceutical Research. 2019;**36**:1-20. DOI: 10.1177/1535676019899502

[38] Navarro SA, Carrillo E, Griñán-Lisón C, Martín A, Perán M, Marchal JA, et al. Cancer suicide gene therapy: A patent review. Expert opinion on therapeutic patents. 2016;**26**(9):1095-1104. DOI: 10.1080/13543776.2016.1211640

[39] Russ E, Iordanskiy S. Endogenous retroviruses as modulators of innate immunity. Pathogens. 2023;**12**(2):162. DOI: 10.3390/pathogens12020162

[40] Hughes SH. Reverse transcription of retroviruses and LTR retrotransposons. Mobile DNA III. 2015;**30**:1051-1077. DOI: 10.1128/microbiolspec.MDNA3-0027-2014

[41] Brommel CM, Cooney AL, Sinn PL. Adeno-associated virus-based gene therapy for lifelong correction of genetic disease. Human Gene Therapy. 2020;**31**(17-18):985-995. DOI: 10.1080/14712598.2020.1725469

[42] Olbrich H, Slabik C, Stripecke R. Reconstructing the immune system with lentiviral vectors. Virus Genes. 2017;**53**(5):723-732. DOI: 10.1007/s11262-017-1495-2

[43] Verhoeyen E, Cosset FL. A3-7 novel lentiviral vector pseudotypes for stable gene transfer into resting hematopoietic cells. In: The Clinic Book. EDP Sciences; 2022. pp. 160-182. DOI: 10.1051/978-2-84254-237-5.c024

[44] Brass AL, Huang IC, Benita Y, John SP, Krishnan MN, Feeley EM, et al. The IFITM proteins mediate cellular resistance to influenza a H1N1 virus, West Nile virus, and dengue virus. Cell. 2009;**139**(7):1243-1254. DOI: 10.1016/j.cell.2009.12.017

[45] Rafiq S, Hackett CS, Brentjens RJ. Engineering strategies to overcome the current roadblocks in CAR T cell therapy. Nature reviews Clinical oncology. 2020;**17**(3):147-167. DOI: 10.1038/s41571-019-0297-y

[46] Xia H, Qin M, Wang Z, Wang Y, Chen B, Wan F, et al. A pH−/enzyme-responsive nanoparticle selectively targets endosomal toll-like receptors to potentiate robust cancer vaccination. Nano Letters. 2022;**22**(7):2978-2987. DOI: 10.1021/acs.nanolett.2c00185

[47] Alagoz M, Kherad N. Advance genome editing technologies in the treatment of human diseases: CRISPR therapy review. International Journal of Molecular Medicine. 2020;**46**(2):521-534. DOI: 10.3892/ijmm.2020.4609

[48] Rubeis G, Steger F. Risks and benefits of human germline genome editing: An ethical analysis. Asian Bioethics Review. 2018;**10**(2):133-141. DOI: 10.1007/s41649-018-0056-x

[49] Uddin F, Rudin CM, Sen T. CRISPR gene therapy: Applications, limitations, and implications for the future. Frontiers in Oncology. 2020;**10**:1387. DOI: 10.3389/fonc.2020.01387

[50] Gregg AR, Skotko BG, Benkendorf JL, Monaghan KG, Bajaj K, Best RG, et al. ACMG noninvasive prenatal screening work group. Noninvasive prenatal screening for fetal aneuploidy, 2016 update: A position statement of the American College of Medical Genetics and Genomics. Genetics in Medicine. 2016;**18**(10):1056-1065. DOI: 10.1038/gim.2016.97

[51] Ormond KE, Mortlock DP, Scholes DT, Bombard Y, Brody LC, Faucett WA, et al. Human germline genome editing. The American Journal of Human Genetics. 2017;**101**(2):167-176. DOI: 10.1016/j.ajhg.2017.06.012

[52] Sadler TD, Zeidler DL. The morality of socioscientific issues: Construal and resolution of genetic engineering dilemmas. Science Education. 2004;**88**(1):4-27. DOI: 10.1002/sce.10101

Chapter 4

HIV Treatment and Obesity: What's New?

Paula Freitas and Sara Ribeiro

Abstract

Obesity among people living with human immunodeficiency virus (people living with human immunodeficiency virus (HIV) (PLWH)) is an emerging public health issue. In recent years, new drugs have been approved for the treatment of HIV infection, which have greatly extended the lives of patients, but they may also play a role in rising obesity rates. In addition to HIV-specific factors, traditional risk factors shared with the general population (aging, diet, inactivity, and genetics) are credible culprits for this pandemic. Importantly, the compounded presence of obesity and HIV infection seems to magnify the risk of metabolic disease. To date, several questions remain to be fully elucidated including the mechanisms by which antiretroviral drugs may lead to excessive weight gain, the influence of the interplay with environmental and genetic factors, and the long-term clinical effect of obesity in PLWH. Recently, new drugs for the treatment of obesity and new metabolic surgeries have emerged, shading new hope on obesity management. The aim of this chapter is to take a journey into the world of obesity, showing the most recent evidence in HIV patients.

Keywords: obesity, human immunodeficiency virus (HIV), antiretroviral therapy, anti-obesity treatments, metabolic surgery

1. Introduction

Infection with the human immunodeficiency virus (HIV) was once a debilitating and ultimately fatal condition. With the advent of highly active antiretroviral therapy (HAART), posteriorly renamed combined antiretroviral therapy (cART), the course of the disease has rapidly changed. HIV is now considered a chronic and manageable condition with a significant improvement in life expectancy, meaning that individuals infected with HIV are at risk of the same comorbidities as an aging population without HIV may suffer, including obesity and its related metabolic dysfunction and cardiovascular disorders [1, 2]. Furthermore, people living with HIV (PLWH) face additional problems as HIV itself is an independent risk factor for metabolic and cardiac disorders, and modern cART regimens may promote excessive weight gain in some HIV-infected patients [3].

Obesity is one of the greatest pandemics of the twenty-first century, and since 1980, its prevalence has doubled in more than 70 countries. Over 600 million adults were obese in 2015, with a high body mass index (BMI) accounting for approximately 4 million deaths worldwide and several years of lost lifespan [4, 5].

Obesity is a chronic, complex, heterogeneous, and relapsing disease that remains a global health concern, associated with an increased risk of multiple conditions [6].

In HIV-infected patients, the presence of obesity may potentially increase the risk of morbidity and mortality. Hence, it is crucial to promptly act to prevent and/or treat obesity in PLWH, paying special attention to the potential impact of antiretroviral therapy on weight gain [7].

The treatment of obesity is challenging and frequently requires a multidisciplinary approach including lifestyle modifications, behavioral therapy, pharmacotherapy, and/or bariatric surgery. In recent years, new drugs have been approved (with others underway) that are revolutionizing the way obesity is treated and will be treated in the near future [8].

Much of the knowledge about pharmacological obesity treatment is extrapolated from studies in people without HIV, but a growing body of research has come to light in recent years regarding nonpharmacological and pharmacological treatment and bariatric surgery in HIV-infected patients [9, 10].

The aim of this chapter is to provide an overview of the pathophysiology, impact, and management of obesity in the context of HIV infection, highlighting the most recent advances on the field.

2. Pathophysiology of obesity in people living with HIV

Following the widespread trend of rising obesity rates and thanks to the undisputable success of cART in prolonging the life expectancy of PLWH, obesity in PLWH is also becoming an emerging public health challenge. In recent years, the prevalence of obesity among PLWH in high-income countries has risen and is now estimated to be 12.5–34% [7, 11, 12]; the same trend is found in low-middle-income countries [13, 14].

Obesity is associated with increased adipose tissue, a special connective tissue containing adipocytes and several other types of cells, surrounded by capillary and innervation networks that function together as an integrated unit. In addition to the classical functions attributed to adipose tissue such as lipid storage, thermal activity, and mechanical insulation, this tissue is also now recognized as a multifunctional and metabolically active immune and endocrine organ, directly modulating many processes including energy balance and metabolism [15].

In obesity, dysfunctional adipocytes and resident-immune cells, particularly T cells and macrophages, display distinct biochemical properties with a pro-inflammatory profile and altered secretion of adipokines and lipokines, thereby creating and perpetuating a state of chronic inflammation, which contributes to the development of comorbidities such as insulin resistance and type 2 diabetes mellitus (T2DM), atherosclerosis, and nonalcoholic fatty liver disease (nonalcoholic steatohepatitis NASH) [16]. Among PLWH, a high BMI has also been shown to magnify the risk of metabolic disease and neurocognitive impairment [17–19]. In fact, HIV-infected patients are a particularly high-risk group, as HIV infection per se, even when treated, induces a state of chronic inflammation and immune activation that contributes to the development of metabolic disease [20]. Accordingly, HIV and obesity seem to act synergistically enhancing the risk of T2DM, as demonstrated in a study that included 7177 HIV-positive American veterans in which a 5-pound gain was associated with a 14% increased risk for diabetes in HIV-infected compared with only 8% in the general population [21].

The anatomical distribution of fat also influences its pro-inflammatory properties. Depending on where it is localized, adipose tissue can be classified as subcutaneous,

DOI: http://dx.doi.org/10.5772/intechopen.112667

with peripheral distribution, or visceral adipose tissue, mainly present in the mesentery and omentum. Clinically, visceral adipose tissue may be evaluated by measures such as increased waist circumference or waist-to-hip ratio, as well as elevated intra-abdominal fat area in cross-sectional abdominal imaging. Visceral adipose tissue has distinct physiological and prognostic differences in comparison with subcutaneous fat, being more cellular, vascular, innervated, and containing a higher number of inflammatory and immune cells [22]. In accordance with these features, visceral adipose tissue is strongly associated with increased cardiometabolic risk and carries a greater prediction of mortality than subcutaneous adipose tissue.

In fact, evidence suggests that the quantity of visceral fat may dictate whether an individual has a "metabolically healthy obesity" (obesity without overt metabolic disease) or a metabolically unhealthy obesity (with metabolic syndrome) [15]. This also seems to hold true in PLWH. In a study that included 580 HIV-infected patients, the proportion of "metabolically unhealthy" patients (patients with metabolic syndrome) was higher among patients with excessive weight and central obesity, with those patients presenting a higher cardiovascular risk [23]. This highlights the importance of addressing obesity and its phenotype (visceral adipose tissue vs. subcutaneous adipose tissue) in patients with HIV, when evaluating cardiometabolic risk [23].

Despite many years of research, the etiopathogenesis of obesity remains to be completely elucidated. Although simple in its most basic principle—it results from an energetic imbalance in which the caloric intake exceeds ongoing energy expenditure—growing evidence indicates that obesity pathogenesis involves processes far more complex than the passive accumulation of excess calories [24]. Many elements influence this equation including genetic, behavioral, and environmental factors, the sleep-wake cycle, hormonal changes, intestinal microbiota, stress, endocrine diseases, and drugs [25]. Besides the antiretroviral agents, many other drugs are also associated with weight gain including antidiabetic agents (insulin, meglitinides, sulfonylureas, and thiazolidinediones), neurologic agents (anticonvulsants, lithium), psychiatric agents [selective serotonin reuptake inhibitors (SSRIs), tricyclic antidepressants (TCAs), antipsychotics, monoamine oxidase inhibitors (MAOIs), and phenothiazines], and other agents (α-adrenergic blockers, antihistamines, β-adrenergic blockers, centrally acting agents, corticosteroids, and hormonal contraceptives) [26].

Sedentary lifestyle, influences of cultural dietary practices, and lack of education or resources regarding proper nutrition are primary drivers for significant weight gain [10]. In addition to quantity, diet quality also determines the obesogenic effects of foods and affects metabolic health through diverse biological pathways [27]. In this regard, increasing attention is being paid to food insecurity and its role in obesity.

3. Food insecurity in PLWH

Food insecurity is defined as having limited or uncertain access to nutritionally adequate and safe foods to maintain a healthy life [28].

Likely a consequence of the socioeconomic challenges that many HIV-infected patients experience, PLWH are disproportionately affected by food insecurity with studies suggesting that up to half of PLWH in urban areas of North America experience food insecurity [29].

Food insecurity is a known risk factor for obesity in both PLWH and HIV-uninfected people [30] and is a major determinant of poor nutrition; PLWH with food insecurity can have a similar caloric intake as people with food security, but of poorer quality based on nutrient-poor, energy-dense food [31–33]. Very low food security has been associated with more frequent frailty among women, independently of HIV serostatus and has been implicated in worse clinical outcomes in PLWH, the reason why it should be part of the assessment in PLWH and obesity [33].

In conclusion, obesity is an emerging comorbidity in PLWH with important metabolic consequences. Several factors are implicated, many of which are shared with HIV-uninfected patients, such as diet and sedentarism. However, PLWH face the additional burden of obesity-promoting HIV-specific factors, notably the overlapping immune activation arising from chronic HIV infection and exposure to antiretroviral therapy (ART).

4. The new era of antiretroviral therapy: integrase inhibitors

In the early days of the HIV epidemic and cART, weight gain in PLWH, particularly in those with low CD4 count and high HIV RNA, was attributed to the reversal of the catabolic state of HIV infection and was associated with improved survival and immunologic recovery, and therefore was considered a "return to health" [34]. Back in those days, the major concern regarding fat alterations was lipodystrophy, characterized by subcutaneous fat loss (lipoatrophy) with or without central fat accumulation. Lipodystrophy was a frequent condition among PLWH receiving combination antiretroviral therapy containing older-generation thymidine analog nucleoside reverse transcriptase inhibitors (NRTIs) and early protease inhibitors (PIs) [35]. In the last 20 years, however, the scenario has changed. Greatly thanks to an earlier diagnosis and highly effective newer generation cART, wasting syndrome and lipodystrophy have become much rarer. Instead, weight gain and obesity are becoming the greatest concern as evidence coming from a multitude of studies show that the median BMI and prevalence of baseline obesity among PLWH initiating cART have been steadily increasing, with most of the patients having normal or high BMI [36]. Moreover, following cART initiation many individuals gain an excessive amount of weight, leading to posttreatment obesity. In a study by Tate and colleagues in 2012, 20% of PLWH had moved to a more deleterious BMI category (from normal to overweight/obese or overweight to obese BMI categories) after 24 months on cART, with greater BMI increases observed for those on a boosted protease inhibitor (PI) regimen [37].

In line with these results, the North America AIDS Cohort Collaboration on Research and Design (NA-ACCORD) study that included over 14,000 individuals showed that after 3 years on cART, 22% of individuals with a normal BMI at baseline had become overweight (BMI 25–29.9 kg/m^2) and 18% of those overweight at baseline had become obese (BMI >30 kg/m^2). The weight gain was largest for women and, for White women greater than age-matched population control [36].

The same phenomenon seems to be replicated and aggravated with newer ART regimens as accumulating evidence suggests that therapies including new generation integrase strand transfer inhibitors (INSTIs) cause more weight gain and treatment-emergent obesity than other ART regimens [38–41].

The first INSTI approved by the U.S. Food and Drug Administration (FDA) was raltegravir in 2007, followed by approval of five other drugs: raltegravir, elvitegravir, cabotegravir, dolutegravir, and bictegravir. Since 2017, acknowledging the good tolerability profile and (for the latter two), a substantial genetic barrier to drug resistance, the INSTI integrate the preferred combination of antiretroviral drugs for initial therapy (consisting of two nucleoside reverse transcriptase inhibitors (NRTIs) and an INSTI) [42].

From 2006 to 2019, the Women's Interagency HIV Study enrolled a geographically and racially diverse sample of 1458 women living HIV and on ART. In this relevant sample, the switch from non-INSTI regimens to INSTIs and/or tenofovir alafenamide (TAF) was associated with significant short-term body weight and BMI gains [43]. Additionally, results from five randomized studies support the association between the use of INSTIs and increases in weight (two studies evaluated raltegravir and three evaluated dolutegravir) [44].

The statistically significant increases in body weight and clinical obesity with INSTIs appear to be most pronounced in Black individuals and women, suggesting the presence of vulnerable subgroups. The effect of cART drugs on weight gain is heterogeneous and differences clearly exist among various INSTIs and NRTI backbones; in particular, evidence suggests that tenofovir alafenamide (TAF) potentially enhances the weight gain effect and that the use of tenofovir disoproxil fumarate (TDF) seems to lessen these effects [44]. In what respects INSTIs and dolutegravir appear to have the greatest effect, while elvitegravir may have minimal effect. Evidence on cabotegravir, the newest integrase inhibitor, is limited [45]. Novel treatments such as the next-generation NNRTI doravirine could offer a suitable alternative therapy, with current evidence showing efficacy and limited effect on weight gain [39].

Still, data on this topic are inconsistent, and more randomized studies accounting for diet and lifestyle factors, such as smoking, are needed. It remains unclear whether INSTI-based regimens also contribute to visceral adiposity or intensification of the cardiometabolic risk [46].

The mechanisms driving weight gain following cART remain largely unknown and certainly override the traditional concept of "return to health." Proposed mechanisms include improved tolerability, direct impact on adipogenesis, and gut microbiome disturbance [39, 45]. Alterations in the composition and function of the intestinal microbiome seem to precede weight gain and may promote obesity through increased bowel permeability, increased fermentation and absorption of dietary polysaccharides, and even through modulation of genes regulating lipogenesis and insulin resistance [47].

Furthermore, *in vitro* studies have shown that dolutegravir inhibits the binding of radiolabeled α-melanocyte-stimulating hormone (MSH) to the human recombinant melanocortin 4 (MC4R) [48]. Since MC4R is involved in the regulation of energy homeostasis and food intake, and deficiency in MC4R is associated with monogenic obesity, increased appetite caused by dolutegravir could contribute to the observed changes [49].

5. Treatment of obesity

Many strategies can be effective in inducing weight loss in people with obesity, including low-calorie diets, exercise-based interventions, pharmacological treatments, and surgery, either separately or in combination [50]. Besides the beneficial impact on weight, these interventions also lead to enhanced quality of life in addition to improvement in glycemic and lipid control, particularly for those who lose more than 10% of their baseline weight [50, 51]. However, how weight loss exactly affects adipose tissue physiology and obesity-related systemic inflammation as well as its long-term implications in terms of mortality and life expectancy remain to be fully clarified [52].

In PLWH specifically, obesity treatment remains largely unaddressed and little research has yet tested the efficacy of these weight loss programs and whether the benefits translate to this population.

Understanding the multifactorial nature of obesity is essential for better informing its management [38].

6. Nonpharmacological treatment

When determining the optimal weight-loss strategy for individuals living with HIV (PLWH), several factors should be considered.

Lifestyle interventions are crucial in addressing obesity and typically encompass a combination of dietary modifications, physical activity, and behavioral strategies. Caloric restriction should be contemplated as the primary element in weight-loss interventions. Additionally, aerobic exercise and resistance training are recommended for all individuals [53]. Behavioral interventions also play a pivotal role in obesity management; strategies, such as self-monitoring, goal-setting, stress management, and social support systems, can enhance adherence to lifestyle changes and improve long-term outcomes [54].

The optimal lifestyle approach for weight loss in PLWH has not yet been defined. For example, multiple interventions, such as low-fat, Mediterranean, or micronutrient-supplemented nutrition, combined with behavioral interventions, have shown modest improvements in blood pressure, metabolic parameters, immune activation, and favorable gut microbiota changes [55–59]. However, these studies were mainly designed to target cardiovascular factors and/or lipodystrophy rather than on weight loss and its long-term maintenance.

In general, when studied in those without HIV, the effect of different dietary macronutrient patterns (carbohydrate reduction, fat reduction, and moderate macronutrients) and popular named diet programs on weight loss has found small differences of limited clinical significance [60]. Although a recent meta-analysis showed that most macronutrient diets lead to modest weight reductions and substantial improvements in blood pressure and lipids over 6 months, the effects were not sustained [61]. On the other hand, higher intakes of protein and fiber, as well as lower glycemic load diets, seem to contribute to weight maintenance by increasing satiety [62]. The Mediterranean diet has been shown to improve metabolic parameters, immune activation, regulatory T-cell (Treg) function, and the composition of the gut microbiota in HIV-1-infected individuals. Furthermore, the Mediterranean diet has been associated with increased abundances of *Bifidobacterium* after the intervention, which is linked to a beneficial profile [58]. Data are still lacking regarding the effects of intermittent fasting regimens in PLWH with obesity and directed clinical trials are warranted [63].

When addressing obesity, it is crucial to set a realistic and meaningful weight goal. People can lose weight on any dietary plan as long as a total caloric deficit is achieved. The choice of a dietary approach should be individualized, but typically, a deficit of at least 500 kcal per day can lead to a loss of 0.5–1.0 kg per week. Sustained weight loss of as little as 3–5% of body weight can result in clinically meaningful reductions in specific risk factors associated with cardiovascular disease (CVD) [64]. Moreover, moderate diet-induced weight loss (6–8%) has been shown to improve metabolic function in people with HIV, obesity, and insulin resistance [65].

7. Physical activity and exercise training

Compared to adults without HIV but with other chronic diseases, PLWH generally tend to be less physically active [66], which may contribute to weight gain. Studies

DOI: http://dx.doi.org/10.5772/intechopen.112667

investigating the benefits of combined aerobic and resistance exercise training in PLWH have consistently shown (despite the relatively small sample sizes and short intervention duration) physiological improvements, including lower BMI, waist circumference, improved lipid profile, and enhanced cardiorespiratory fitness [67]. Additionally, exercise has been associated with reduced distress, lower levels of depression, and improved neurocognitive function [68–71].

As a principle, PLHW should follow the general guidelines that recommend engaging in 30 min or more of moderate-intensity physical activity most days of the week for weight loss and maintenance, with the goal of achieving a minimum of 150 min per week [64, 67]. Resistance training should also be incorporated into the regimen, preferably performed 2 to 3 times per week [53]. Furthermore, periodization of exercise, which involves manipulating the volume, intensity, and recovery between exercises, has also demonstrated better results than nonperiodized training in PLWH [72] and can be considered.

In conclusion, exercise training is considered safe and beneficial for medically stable adults living with HIV and should be part of the recommendations [68].

8. Metabolic adaptation

Why do people who follow a diet plan not continue to lose weight? And why is weight regain so common? The answer lies in metabolic adaptation.

Metabolic adaptation occurs during weight loss and involves an increase in hunger as a result of elevated levels of the orexigenic hormone ghrelin and decreased levels of anorexigenic hormones. Simultaneously, energy requirements decrease, thereby creating what is known as the "energy gap" [62]. The decrease in total daily energy expenditure that occurs during weight loss results from many contributors such as a decrease in circulating leptin levels, a reduction in resting metabolic rate, a diminished thermic effect of food, and increased energy efficiency during daily activities [62]. Further investigation is required to identify effective strategies for narrowing the energy gap and reducing weight regain. Nevertheless, factors related to long-term weight loss maintenance have been recognized and include increased protein and dietary fiber intake, consuming diets with lower glycemic loads, and high levels of physical activity. Maintaining a high-energy flux state, characterized by a significant daily energy expenditure that matches energy intake, may help mitigate reductions in resting metabolic rate and may facilitate a more precise regulation of energy intake to align with daily energy expenditure [62].

9. Pharmacological treatment of obesity

Limited information is available regarding the safety and effectiveness of weight-loss medications in PLWH since they are often excluded from clinical trials and not adequately reported. However, the efficacy of treatment is likely to be similar to that in the general population, although potential interactions with antiretroviral therapy need to be considered. Notably, there are theoretical and documented drug-drug interactions between anti-obesity pharmacotherapy and antiretroviral therapy [10]. Therefore, healthcare providers must acknowledge the potential hazard of impaired control over HIV viremia when specific weight-loss medications are administered concurrently with antiretroviral therapy [10].

Glucagon-like peptide 1 (GLP-1) receptor agonists have demonstrated promising results in managing obesity in individuals without HIV, and studies investigating their effectiveness in PLWH are currently underway.

Further research is needed to optimize the selection of ART and the combined use of weight loss medications, when indicated [38].

10. Orlistat

Orlistat is the sole anti-obesity drug approved by the FDA and European Medicines Agency (EMA) available both as a prescription medication and an over-the-counter (OTC) product. This accessibility allows widespread public use without close medical supervision [10].

Orlistat induces weight loss by reversibly inhibiting the activity of the enzyme lipase and consequently blocking the hydrolysis of triglycerides into absorbable fatty acids and monoglycerides. Hence, orlistat acts mainly via its local effect, directly reducing the absorption of dietary fat by around 30% [10]. Systemic exposure is minimal as it is primarily metabolized within the gastrointestinal wall and mostly undergoes fecal elimination. While orlistat does not interfere with the activity or elimination of other drugs through conventional mechanisms, it can potentially interact with other medications due to its impact on absorption [10, 73].

The impact of orlistat on weight loss, weight maintenance, cardiovascular disease risk, and glycemic control has undergone thorough investigation among overweight individuals, including those with and without T2DM. In the Xenical in the Prevention of Diabetes in Obese Subjects (XENDOS) study, participants who received orlistat, in addition to lifestyle changes, experienced an average weight change of 5.8 kg throughout the study duration, compared to a mean weight change of 3 kg in the lifestyle plus placebo group ($p < 0.001$). Furthermore, orlistat therapy reduced the incidence of T2DM beyond the result obtained with lifestyle changes only, an effect particularly evident in patients with impaired glucose tolerance at baseline [74]. Notably, while clinical trials have not explicitly excluded individuals with HIV infection, there is a lack of data specifically documenting outcomes in this particular population [10].

Regarding the safety of orlistat use in PLWH, multiple case reports have linked the initiation of this weight-loss agent to loss of HIV viremia control [10].

In general, drugs classified as Class II according to the Biopharmaceutics Drug Disposition Classification System (BDDCS), characterized by extensive metabolism, low water solubility, and high lipid permeability, are prone to significant alterations when-coadministered with orlistat, potentially resulting in unfavorable outcomes [10].

Significantly, non-nucleoside reverse transcriptase inhibitors (NNRTIs), protease inhibitors (PIs), and integrase inhibitors (INSTIs) are classified as BDDCS Class II drugs, which imply that coadministration with orlistat is likely to result in reduced drug absorption [10]. Furthermore, NRTis, such as zidovudine, abacavir, and TDF, although belonging to different BDDCS classes, are generally acknowledged to possess lipophilic properties [75–77], hence enhancing the probability of potential interferences. Considering the significant risk associated with compromised control of HIV viremia, the absence of efficacy data in HIV patients, and the availability of alternative weight-loss agents suitable for PLWH, orlistat is generally not recommended in all HIV patients currently taking cART. Given the over-the-counter (OTC) availability of orlistat, it is critical that PLWH on cART are properly advised to consult their health-care provider before independently initiating any weight-loss medication [10].

DOI: http://dx.doi.org/10.5772/intechopen.112667

11. Naltrexone-bupropion

Naltrexone-bupropion is a combination regimen that consists of an opioid antagonist (naltrexone) and an aminoketone antidepressant (bupropion). The use of bupropion in combination with naltrexone is believed to help regulate food intake by leveraging their individual effects on the mesolimbic dopamine circuit and hypothalamus, respectively.

In phase 3 trials, such as Contrave Obesity Research-I (COR-I), Contrave Obesity Research-II (COR-II), Contrave Obesity Research-Intensive Behavior Modification (COR-BMOD), and Contrave Obesity Research-Diabetes study (COR-Diabetes), the administration of naltrexone-bupropion demonstrated significant weight reduction compared to placebo [78–81]. Using a modified intent-to-treat analysis, these trials reported average weight losses of approximately 4.7, 5.9, 4.2, and 3.4 kg, respectively, surpassing the outcomes observed with placebo [82]. However, it is important to note that these trials did not include individuals with HIV [10].

Naltrexone and its major active metabolite, 6-β-naltrexol, undergo minimal metabolism by cytochrome P450 (CYP) enzymes and do not exhibit significant inhibition or induction capabilities. Both the parent compound and metabolite are primarily eliminated through renal excretion, with average elimination half-lives of 4 and 13 h, respectively [83].

In contrast, bupropion undergoes extensive hepatic metabolism via cytochrome P450 2B6 (CYP 2B6) to hydroxybupropion, while non-CYP-mediated pathways contribute to the production of erythrohydrobupropion and threohydrobupropion. Bupropion has an average half-life of 21 h, whereas its metabolites exhibit extended half-life in comparison with the parent compound [10].

Based on the pharmacokinetics of bupropion, multiple drug-drug interactions can be recognized or anticipated. Importantly, antiretroviral agents, such as ritonavir and certain NNRTIs, are known inducers of CYP2B6, which may potentially interfere with bupropion concentration. However, at present, no dose adjustments are recommended based on the current understanding of this interaction.

Still, for healthcare providers considering the initiation of naltrexone-bupropion in PLWH, increased monitoring of bupropion is recommended when coadministration with ritonavir-boosted PIs, efavirenz, nevirapine, or any regimen containing cobicistat is planned. Periodic monitorization should include evaluating the efficacy of weight loss, assessing the occurrence of neuropsychiatric events and suicidal behavior and ideation, and evaluating blood pressure, heart rate, and renal and hepatic function. In the event of negative changes in mood or behavior, irrespective of the HIV status or antiretroviral regimen, it is recommended to promptly initiate a tapering process and discontinue the use of naltrexone-buproprion for all patients [10].

12. Liraglutide

Liraglutide is a GLP-1 receptor analog primarily designed for treating T2DM. It is administered via subcutaneous injection and is highly bound to human serum albumin, with more than 99% binding *in vitro*. Liraglutide promotes weight loss by slowing gastric emptying and inducing early satiety [84, 85].

The efficacy of liraglutide for weight loss in patients without T2DM was evaluated in the Satiety and Clinical Adiposity–Liraglutide Evidence (SCALE) randomized controlled clinical trial. In this study, 3.0 mg of liraglutide in addition to diet and exercise was associated with a significant reduction in body weight (mean weight change of 8.4 kg compared to a mean weight change of 2.8 kg with placebo, at week 56 of treatment) [86]. However, individuals living with HIV were not eligible for enrollment in this trial. Other studies, primarily conducted to address liraglutide efficacy in treating T2DM although not explicitly excluding PLWH, have not conducted specific subgroup analysis on this patient population [10]. Nevertheless, based on what it is currently known, there is no reason to expect the benefits of liraglutide therapy in PLWH to differ from the general population.

Liraglutide undergoes rapid clearance by the kidneys through metabolism by endogenous dipeptidyl peptidase IV (DPP-IV) and endopeptidases [87]. As it undergoes a metabolism pathway independent of CYP, the potential for drug-drug interactions is greatly reduced, simplifying its use in individuals receiving cART. Nonetheless, concerns have been raised regarding interactions between liraglutide and antiretroviral agents that necessitate an acidic gastric environment for proper absorption, due to the known inhibitory effect of the natural GLP-1 hormone on gastric secretion. However, an evaluation of individuals at steady state using liraglutide 1.8 mg compared to placebo reported no statistically or clinically significant differences in gastric pH [88]. Liraglutide was also found to have minimal impact on the gastric absorption of concomitant medications from various Biopharmaceutics Drug Disposition Classification System (BDDCS) classes [88].

Overall, liraglutide is regarded as a viable choice for promoting weight loss in PLWH [10].

13. Semaglutide and tirzepatide

Semaglutide, also a GLP-1 receptor agonist, and tirzepatide, a dual GLP-1/gastric inhibitory peptide (GIP) agonist, are both promising options for weight management.

In the STEP 1 trial, individuals treated with semaglutide achieved an average weight loss of almost 15% from baseline (compared to 2.4% with placebo), and nearly 70% of participants experienced more than a 10% reduction in weight (compared to 10% with placebo) [89]. Recent evidence suggests that tirzepatide demonstrates similar or possibly even superior efficacy compared to semaglutide for weight management [90, 91]. Currently, there are two ongoing clinical trials assessing the safety and efficacy of semaglutide in individuals living with HIV (PWH) who also have obesity, with a focus on weight loss achieved through a combination of semaglutide treatment and diet and exercise interventions. These trials aim to evaluate the effectiveness of semaglutide specifically in PWH and its potential impact on weight reduction compared to diet and exercise alone [92], and its effects on ectopic fat, insulin resistance, inflammation markers, and cardiovascular risk [93].

Importantly, despite the lack of substantial data regarding the impact of GLP-1 receptor analogs on weight-loss in PLWH, initial observational studies indicate that treatment of patients with both HIV infection and T2DM using GLP-1 receptor analogs may provide a protective effect against major adverse cardiovascular events such as myocardial infarction and acute heart failure [94].

Regarding weight-loss drugs currently available in Europe, the majority of drugs are generally considered safe for PLWH undergoing cART, except for orlistat. When planning to start pharmacological treatment for obesity, clinicians should contemplate each agent's specific characteristics, counseling points, and monitoring parameters that necessitate assessment when used in conjunction with cART.

In conclusion, obesity in PLWH should be addressed using a similar approach employed to the general population. Healthcare providers should consider incorporating most of the currently approved weight-loss agents as adjuncts to adequate lifestyle modifications [10].

14. New hopes in the treatment of obesity

Several upcoming drugs promise to revolutionize the treatment of obesity by combining different incretin pathways. Retatrutide (LY3437943), a triple agonist of the glucose-dependent insulinotropic polypeptide, glucagon-like peptide 1, and glucagon receptors, seems of special interest due to the substantial reduction in body weight observed in its Phase 2 trial [95].

Similarly, the coadministration of cagrilintide—a long-acting amylin analogue—and semaglutide (CagriSema), resulted in clinically relevant improvements in glycemic control and significantly greater weight loss versus semaglutide in people with T2DM [96, 97].

Finally, orforglipron, a nonpeptide GLP-1 receptor agonist given as an once-daily oral therapy, has also shown to lead to substantial weight reduction in adults with obesity without T2M [98]. Phase 3 trials are currently underway for all these new promising drugs. Their role in obesity treatment in PLWH remains to be clarified.

15. Bariatric or metabolic surgery

Bariatric surgery is gaining popularity as an effective surgical intervention for addressing severe obesity and metabolic dysregulation in cases where lifestyle modifications are insufficient to attaining weight-related objectives [99]. Bariatric surgery may be a suitable option for patients with a BMI of 40 kg/m^2 or greater, or a BMI of 35 kg/m^2 or greater with one or more severe obesity-related comorbidities [53]. Given the rising prevalence of obesity in PLWH, bariatric surgery is increasingly being used among PLWH [45].

The American Society for Metabolic and Bariatric Surgery recommends laparoscopic approaches, such as Roux-en-Y gastric bypass, sleeve gastrectomy, adjustable gastric banding, and biliopancreatic diversion/duodenal switch, as preferred methods compared to over open bariatric procedures [99].

There is limited literature available on the efficacy of bariatric surgery in HIV-infected individuals and no large-scale or randomized clinical trials have been conducted in this patient population. However, existing literature suggest that patients with HIV are likely to share the same benefits in terms of weight loss and resolution of obesity-associated comorbidities to those without HIV. Also, data concerning HIV-related outcomes and pharmacokinetics of cART following bariatric surgery remain scarce and, as a result, there are no specific guidelines for managing HIV-infected individuals after bariatric surgery.

Understandably, factors specific to these patients, such as viral load, CD4 cell counts, absorption of antiretroviral therapy, and other medications, are important outcomes to consider [9].

Patients who undergo bariatric surgery experience significant anatomical and physiological alterations, including changes in gastric volume, acidity, gastrointestinal emptying time, enterohepatic circulation, and delayed entry of bile acids [45].

Additionally, they will have to undertake a specific diet plan, may receive instructions to crush oral medications, and may be prescribed postoperative acid-suppressing agents and vitamin supplements. These alterations can affect different aspects of antiretroviral absorption and pharmacokinetics. Some antiretrovirals with specific characteristics, such as requiring an acidic environment, administration with fatty meals, longer intestinal exposure, and enterohepatic recirculation for absorption, may be more impacted by bariatric surgery interventions [45]. Additionally, certain antiretrovirals can interact with polyvalent cations in supplements or drugs that inhibit gastric acid.

In this context, healthcare providers need to carefully evaluate the patient's antiretroviral medications taking into consideration factors such as the absorption site of the antiretrovirals, their compatibility with being crushed, the need for administration with food, and any contraindications or drug interactions with acid-suppressing agents or supplements [99].

Predicting pharmacokinetics based solely on drug characteristics has proven to be challenging, underscoring the importance of pharmacokinetic studies in this specific population [45]. Still, dolutegravir, darunavir, and most NRTIs seem appropriate drug options postbariatric surgery [45] and despite these concerns regarding drug absorption after bariatric surgery, so far, there is no evidence suggesting a significant impact on markers of HIV disease progression, such as CD4 count and viral load, for both sleeve gastrectomy and Roux-en-Y gastric bypass [9, 100, 101].

Finally, recent research has demonstrated that bariatric surgery induces an immediate and enduring modification of the gut microbiota, which is independent of the surgical procedure itself [102]. It has been suggested that changes in the gut microbiome can influence the pharmacokinetics of certain antiretrovirals, such as abacavir and dolutegravir [103]. Gut microbiota alterations can lead to increased levels of s-glucuronidase enzymes in the gut environment, potently increasing the regeneration of active forms of these drugs and resulting in higher exposure concentrations [104]. However, it is important to interpret these data with caution, as the gut microbiome is influenced by multiple interfering factors such as diet, antibiotic use, and demographic parameters, possibly introducing different biases.

In conclusion, bariatric surgery is a viable option for selected patients with obesity, considering its success in driving weight loss without significantly interfering with cART-induced viral suppression. Nevertheless, the potential impact of perioperative changes in diet, supplements, and medications on antiretroviral regimens must always be carefully considered and close surveillance should be maintained [99].

16. Conclusions

Obesity in individuals with HIV is an emergent and complex issue with various contributing factors, many of which are still not fully understood. While research on weight gain and obesity in people living with HIV has increased in recent years, much of the knowledge is based on studies conducted in individuals without HIV.

The increasing rates of obesity among PLWH are most likely multifactorial, resulting from the compounded effect of exposure to the obesogenic environment we currently live in and its associated traditional risk factors (e.g., inactivity, diet, and genetics) and HIV-specific factors including HIV-associated systemic inflammation/immune dysregulation and direct cART effects, most particularly with the use of integrase strand transfer inhibitors.

Importantly, weight gain in PLWH confers a greater risk of metabolic disease compared with HIV-negative individuals, highlighting the need to properly prevent and/or manage obesity in this population.

To improve the care of the growing population of people aging with HIV, it is crucial to better understand the mechanisms and clinical implications of cART-mediated weight gain and obesity.

Prospective clinical trials and further research are needed to optimize ART selection, explore the use of weight loss medications, and determine the efficacy and safety of metabolic surgeries. A multidisciplinary approach involving a team of surgeons, endocrinologists, nutritionists, psychologists, HIV providers, and clinical pharmacists is necessary to effectively prevent and treat obesity in people living with HIV.

The coordination and collaboration of interdisciplinary healthcare professionals are essential to ensure optimal outcomes for this unique patient population.

Author details

Paula Freitas[1,2,3]* and Sara Ribeiro[1,2,3]

1 Department of Endocrinology Diabetes and Metabolism, Centro Hospitalar Universitário de São João, Porto, Portugal

2 Faculty of Medicine, Universidade do Porto, Porto, Portugal

3 Instituto de Investigação e Inovação em Saúde, Universidade do Porto, Porto, Portugal

*Address all correspondence to: paula_freitas@sapo.pt

References

[1] Mahy M, Stover J, Stanecki K, Stoneburner R, Tassie JM. Estimating the impact of antiretroviral therapy: Regional and global estimates of life-years gained among adults. Sexually Transmitted Infections. 2010;**86**(Suppl_2):ii67-ii71

[2] Antiretroviral Therapy Cohort Collaboration, Zwahlen M, Harris R, May M, Hogg R, Costagliola D, et al. Mortality of HIV-infected patients starting potent antiretroviral therapy: Comparison with the general population in nine industrialized countries. International Journal of Epidemiology. 2009;**38**(6):1624-1633

[3] Seecheran VK, Giddings SL, Seecheran NA. Acute coronary syndromes in patients with HIV. Coronary Artery Disease. 2017;**28**(2):166-172

[4] Collaborators GBDO, Afshin A, Forouzanfar MH, Reitsma MB, Sur P, Estep K, et al. Health effects of overweight and obesity in 195 countries over 25 years. The New England Journal of Medicine. 2017;**377**(1):13-27

[5] Bhaskaran K, Dos-Santos-Silva I, Leon DA, Douglas IJ, Smeeth L. Association of BMI with overall and cause-specific mortality: A population-based cohort study of 3.6 million adults in the UK. The Lancet Diabetes and Endocrinology. 2018;**6**(12):944-953

[6] Pi-Sunyer X. The medical risks of obesity. Postgraduate Medicine. 2009;**121**(6):21-33

[7] Yuh B, Tate J, Butt AA, Crothers K, Freiberg M, Leaf D, et al. Weight change after antiretroviral therapy and mortality. Clinical Infectious Diseases. 2015;**60**(12):1852-1859

[8] Chakhtoura M, Haber R, Ghezzawi M, Rhayem C, Tcheroyan R, Mantzoros CS. Pharmacotherapy of obesity: An update on the available medications and drugs under investigation. EClinicalMedicine. 2023;**58**:101882

[9] Akbari K, Som R, Sampson M, Abbas SH, Ramus J, Jones G. The effect of bariatric surgery on patients with HIV infection: A literature review. Obesity Surgery. 2018;**28**(8):2550-2559

[10] Cope RJ, Fischetti BS, Kavanagh RK, Lepa TM, Sorbera MA. Safety and efficacy of weight-loss pharmacotherapy in persons living with HIV: A review of the literature and potential drug-drug interactions with antiretroviral therapy. Pharmacotherapy. 2019;**39**(12):1204-1215

[11] Becofsky KM, Wing EJ, Wing RR, Richards KE, Gillani FS. Obesity prevalence and related risk of comorbidities among HIV+ patients attending a New England ambulatory centre. Obesity Science and Practice. 2016;**2**(2):123-127

[12] Freitas P, Carvalho D, Santos AC, Matos MJ, Madureira AJ, Marques R, et al. Prevalence of obesity and its relationship to clinical lipodystrophy in HIV-infected adults on anti-retroviral therapy. Journal of Endocrinological Investigation. 2012;**35**(11):964-970

[13] Guehi C, Badje A, Gabillard D, Ouattara E, Koule SO, Moh R, et al. High prevalence of being overweight and obese HIV-infected persons, before and after 24 months on early ART in

the ANRS 12136 temprano trial. AIDS Research and Therapy. 2016;**13**:12

[14] Nalugga EA, Laker E, Nabaggala MS, Ddungu A, Batte C, Piloya T, et al. Prevalence of overweight and obesity and associated factors among people living with HIV attending a tertiary care clinic in Uganda. BMC Nutrition. 2022;**8**(1):107

[15] Guerreiro VA, Carvalho D, Freitas P. Obesity, adipose tissue, and inflammation answered in questions. Journal of Obesity. 2022;**2022**:2252516

[16] Scheja L, Heeren J. The endocrine function of adipose tissues in health and cardiometabolic disease. Nature Reviews. Endocrinology. 2019;**15**(9):507-524

[17] Sattler FR, He J, Letendre S, Wilson C, Sanders C, Heaton R, et al. Abdominal obesity contributes to neurocognitive impairment in HIV-infected patients with increased inflammation and immune activation. Journal of Acquired Immune Deficiency Syndromes. 2015;**68**(3):281-288

[18] Kim DJ, Westfall AO, Chamot E, Willig AL, Mugavero MJ, Ritchie C, et al. Multimorbidity patterns in HIV-infected patients: The role of obesity in chronic disease clustering. Journal of Acquired Immune Deficiency Syndromes. 2012;**61**(5):600-605

[19] Jacobson DL, Tang AM, Spiegelman D, Thomas AM, Skinner S, Gorbach SL, et al. Incidence of metabolic syndrome in a cohort of HIV-infected adults and prevalence relative to the US population (national health and nutrition examination survey). Journal of Acquired Immune Deficiency Syndromes. 2006;**43**(4):458-466

[20] Lake JE, Currier JS. Metabolic disease in HIV infection. The Lancet Infectious Diseases. 2013;**13**(11):964-975

[21] Herrin M, Tate JP, Akgun KM, Butt AA, Crothers K, Freiberg MS, et al. Weight gain and incident diabetes among HIV-infected veterans initiating Antiretroviral Therapy compared with uninfected individuals. Journal of Acquired Immune Deficiency Syndromes. 2016;**73**(2):228-236

[22] Ibrahim MM. Subcutaneous and visceral adipose tissue: Structural and functional differences. Obesity Reviews. 2010;**11**(1):11-18

[23] Neves JS, Guerreiro V, Carvalho D, Serrao R, Sarmento A, Freitas P. Metabolically healthy or metabolically unhealthy obese HIV-infected patients: Mostly a matter of age? Frontiers in Endocrinology (Lausanne). 2018;**9**:681

[24] Schwartz MW, Seeley RJ, Zeltser LM, Drewnowski A, Ravussin E, Redman LM, et al. Obesity pathogenesis: An endocrine society scientific statement. Endocrine Reviews. 2017;**38**(4):267-296

[25] Lecube A, Monereo S, Rubio MA, Martinez-de-Icaya P, Marti A, Salvador J, et al. Prevention, diagnosis, and treatment of obesity. 2016 position statement of the Spanish Society for the Study of obesity. Endocrinología, Diabetes y Nutrición. 2017;**64** (Suppl. 1):15-22

[26] Malone M. Medications associated with weight gain. The Annals of Pharmacotherapy. 2005;**39**(12):2046-2055

[27] Jiao J. The role of nutrition in obesity. Nutrients. 2023;**15**:2556. DOI: 10.3390/nu15112556

[28] Anderson SA. Core indicators of nutritional state for difficult-to-sample populations. The Journal of Nutrition. 1990;**120**(Suppl 11):1559-1600

[29] Bekele T, Globerman J, Watson J, Jose-Boebridge M, Kennedy R, Hambly K, et al. Prevalence and predictors of food insecurity among people living with HIV affiliated with AIDS service organizations in Ontario, Canada. AIDS Care. 2018;**30**(5):663-671

[30] Derose KP, Rios-Castillo I, Fulcar MA, Payan DD, Palar K, Escala L, et al. Severe food insecurity is associated with overweight and increased body fat among people living with HIV in the Dominican Republic. AIDS Care. 2018;**30**(2):182-190

[31] Weiser SD, Sheira LA, Palar K, Kushel M, Wilson TE, Adedimeji A, et al. Mechanisms from food insecurity to worse HIV treatment outcomes in US women living with HIV. AIDS Patient Care and STDs. 2020;**34**(10):425-435

[32] Anema A, Fielden SJ, Shurgold S, Ding E, Messina J, Jones JE, et al. Association between food insecurity and procurement methods among people living with HIV in a high resource setting. PLoS One. 2016;**11**(8):e0157630

[33] Tan JY, Sheira LA, Frongillo EA, Gustafson D, Sharma A, Merenstein D, et al. Food insecurity and frailty among women with and without HIV in the United States: A cross-sectional analysis. Journal of the International AIDS Society. 2021;**24**(6):e25751

[34] Kumar S, Samaras K. The impact of weight gain during HIV treatment on risk of pre-diabetes, diabetes mellitus, cardiovascular disease, and mortality. Frontiers in Endocrinology (Lausanne). 2018;**9**:705

[35] Koethe JR, Lagathu C, Lake JE, Domingo P, Calmy A, Falutz J, et al. HIV and antiretroviral therapy-related fat alterations. Nature Reviews. Disease Primers. 2020;**6**(1):48

[36] Koethe JR, Jenkins CA, Lau B, Shepherd BE, Justice AC, Tate JP, et al. Rising obesity prevalence and weight gain among adults starting antiretroviral therapy in the United States and Canada. AIDS Research and Human Retroviruses. 2016;**32**(1):50-58

[37] Tate T, Willig AL, Willig JH, Raper JL, Moneyham L, Kempf MC, et al. HIV infection and obesity: Where did all the wasting go? Antiviral Therapy. 2012;**17**(7):1281-1289

[38] Parra-Rodriguez L, O'Halloran JA. HIV and obesity: Updates in management strategies. Current Opinion in HIV and AIDS. 2023;**18**(2):68-74

[39] Shah S, Hindley L, Hill A. Are new antiretroviral treatments increasing the risk of weight gain? Drugs. 2021;**81**(3):299-315

[40] Bourgi K, Jenkins CA, Rebeiro PF, Palella F, Moore RD, Altoff KN, et al. Weight gain among treatment-naive persons with HIV starting integrase inhibitors compared to non-nucleoside reverse transcriptase inhibitors or protease inhibitors in a large observational cohort in the United States and Canada. Journal of the International AIDS Society. 2020;**23**(4):e25484

[41] Sax PE, Erlandson KM, Lake JE, McComsey GA, Orkin C, Esser S, et al. Weight gain following initiation of antiretroviral therapy: Risk factors in randomized comparative clinical trials. Clinical Infectious Diseases. 2020;**71**(6):1379-1389

[42] Saag MS, Gandhi RT, Hoy JF, Landovitz RJ, Thompson MA, Sax PE, et al. Antiretroviral drugs for treatment and prevention of HIV infection in adults: 2020 recommendations of the international antiviral society-USA panel. Journal of the American Medical Association. 2020;**324**(16):1651-1669

[43] Lahiri CD, Xu Y, Wang K, Alvarez JA, Sheth AN, O'Halloran J, et al. Weight and body mass index change after switching to integrase inhibitors or Tenofovir Alafenamide among women living with HIV. AIDS Research and Human Retroviruses. 2021;**37**(6):461-467

[44] Hill A, Waters L, Pozniak A. Are new antiretroviral treatments increasing the risks of clinical obesity? Journal of Virus Eradication. 2019;**5**(1):41-43

[45] Zino L, Kingma JS, Marzolini C, Richel O, Burger DM, Colbers A. Implications of bariatric surgery on the pharmacokinetics of antiretrovirals in people living with HIV. Clinical Pharmacokinetics. 2022;**61**(5):619-635

[46] Eckard AR, McComsey GA. Weight gain and integrase inhibitors. Current Opinion in Infectious Diseases. 2020;**33**(1):10-19

[47] Cornejo-Pareja I, Munoz-Garach A, Clemente-Postigo M, Tinahones FJ. Importance of gut microbiota in obesity. European Journal of Clinical Nutrition. 2019;**72**(Suppl 1):26-37

[48] Agency EM. Assessment report. Dolutegravir (Tivicay). 2013. Available from: https://www.ema.europa.eu/en/ documents/assessment-report/tivicayepar-public-assessment-report_en.p

[49] Bourgi K, Rebeiro PF, Turner M, Castilho JL, Hulgan T, Raffanti SP, et al. Greater weight gain in treatment-naive persons starting dolutegravir-based antiretroviral therapy. Clinical Infectious Diseases. 2020;**70**(7):1267-1274

[50] Forsythe LK, Wallace JM, Livingstone MB. Obesity and inflammation: The effects of weight loss. Nutrition Research Reviews. 2008;**21**(2):117-133

[51] Shi Q, Wang Y, Hao Q, Vandvik PO, Guyatt G, Li J, et al. Pharmacotherapy for adults with overweight and obesity: A systematic review and network meta-analysis of randomised controlled trials. Lancet. 2022;**399**(10321):259-269

[52] Savinelli S, Wrigley Kelly NE, Feeney ER, O'Shea DB, Hogan AE, Overton ET, et al. Obesity in HIV infection: Host-pathogen interaction. AIDS. 2022;**36**(11):1477-1491

[53] Garvey WT, Mechanick JI, Brett EM, Garber AJ, Hurley DL, Jastreboff AM, et al. American association of clinical endocrinologists and American college of endocrinology comprehensive clinical practice guidelines for medical care of patients with obesity. Endocrine Practice. 2016;**22**(Suppl. 3):1-203

[54] Olateju IV, Ogwu D, Owolabi MO, Azode U, Osula F, Okeke R, et al. Role of behavioral interventions in the management of obesity. Cureus. 2021;**13**(9):e18080

[55] Panza E, Wing EJ, Wing R. Behavioral weight loss: A promising treatment for obesity in adults with HIV. AIDS and Behavior. 2020;**24**(4):1085-1091

[56] Saumoy M, Alonso-Villaverde C, Navarro A, Olmo M, Vila R, Ramon JM, et al. Randomized trial of a multidisciplinary lifestyle intervention

in HIV-infected patients with moderate-high cardiovascular risk. Atherosclerosis. 2016;**246**:301-308

[57] Webel AR, Moore SM, Longenecker CT, Currie J, Horvat Davey C, Perazzo J, et al. Randomized controlled trial of the SystemCHANGE intervention on behaviors related to cardiovascular risk in HIV+ adults. Journal of Acquired Immune Deficiency Syndromes. 2018;**78**(1):23-33

[58] Pastor-Ibanez R, Blanco-Heredia J, Etcheverry F, Sanchez-Palomino S, Diez-Fuertes F, Casas R, et al. Adherence to a supplemented mediterranean diet drives changes in the gut microbiota of HIV-1-infected individuals. Nutrients. 2021;**13**(4):1141. DOI: 10.3390/nu13041141

[59] Stradling C, Thomas GN, Hemming K, Taylor S, Taheri S. Randomized parallel-group pilot trial (best foods for your heart) comparing the effects of a mediterranean portfolio diet with a low saturated fat diet on HIV dyslipidemia. Clinical Nutrition. 2021;**40**(3):860-869

[60] Johnston BC, Kanters S, Bandayrel K, Wu P, Naji F, Siemieniuk RA, et al. Comparison of weight loss among named diet programs in overweight and obese adults: A meta-analysis. Journal of the American Medical Association. 2014;**312**(9):923-933

[61] Ge L, Sadeghirad B, Ball GDC, da Costa BR, Hitchcock CL, Svendrovski A, et al. Comparison of dietary macronutrient patterns of 14 popular named dietary programmes for weight and cardiovascular risk factor reduction in adults: Systematic review and network meta-analysis of randomised trials. BMJ. 2020;**369**:m696

[62] Melby CL, Paris HL, Foright RM, Peth J. Attenuating the biologic drive for weight regain following weight loss: Must what goes down always go Back up? Nutrients. 2017;**9**:468. DOI: 10.3390/nu9050468

[63] Gnoni M, Beas R, Raghuram A, Diaz-Pardave C, Riva-Moscoso A, Principe-Meneses FS, et al. Potential role of intermittent fasting on decreasing cardiovascular disease in human immunodeficiency virus patients receiving antiretroviral therapy. World Journal of Experimental Medicine. 2021;**11**(5):66-78

[64] Jensen MD, Ryan DH, Apovian CM, Ard JD, Comuzzie AG, Donato KA, et al. 2013 AHA/ACC/TOS guideline for the management of overweight and obesity in adults: A report of the American College of Cardiology/American Heart Association task force on practice guidelines and the obesity society. Circulation. 2014;**129** (25 Suppl. 2):S102-S138

[65] Reeds DN, Pietka TA, Yarasheski KE, Cade WT, Patterson BW, Okunade A, et al. HIV infection does not prevent the metabolic benefits of diet-induced weight loss in women with obesity. Obesity (Silver Spring). 2017;**25**(4):682-688

[66] Vancampfort D, Mugisha J, De Hert M, Probst M, Firth J, Gorczynski P, et al. Global physical activity levels among people living with HIV: A systematic review and meta-analysis. Disability and Rehabilitation. 2018;**40**(4):388-397

[67] Jaggers JR, Hand GA. Health benefits of exercise for people living with HIV: A review of the literature. American Journal of Lifestyle Medicine. 2016;**10**(3):184-192

[68] O'Brien KK, Tynan AM, Nixon SA, Glazier RH. Effectiveness of aerobic

exercise for adults living with HIV: Systematic review and meta-analysis using the Cochrane collaboration protocol. BMC Infectious Diseases. 2016;**16**:182

[69] Fazeli PL, Marquine MJ, Dufour C, Henry BL, Montoya J, Gouaux B, et al. Physical activity is associated with better neurocognitive and everyday functioning among older adults with HIV disease. AIDS and Behavior. 2015;**19**(8):1470-1477

[70] Webel AR, Perazzo J, Decker M, Horvat-Davey C, Sattar A, Voss J. Physical activity is associated with reduced fatigue in adults living with HIV/AIDS. Journal of Advanced Nursing. 2016;**72**(12):3104-3112

[71] Webel AR, Willig AL, Liu W, Sattar A, Boswell S, Crane HM, et al. Physical activity intensity is associated with symptom distress in the CNICS Cohort. AIDS and Behavior. 2019;**23**(3):627-635

[72] Soares VL, Soares WF, Zanetti HR, Neves FF, Silva-Vergara ML, Mendes EL. Daily undulating periodization is more effective than nonperiodized training on maximal strength, aerobic capacity, and TCD4+ cell count in people living with HIV. Journal of Strength and Conditioning Research. 2022;**36**(6):1738-1748

[73] Filippatos TD, Derdemezis CS, Gazi IF, Nakou ES, Mikhailidis DP, Elisaf MS. Orlistat-associated adverse effects and drug interactions: A critical review. Drug Safety. 2008;**31**(1):53-65

[74] Torgerson JS, Hauptman J, Boldrin MN, Sjostrom L. XENical in the prevention of diabetes in obese subjects (XENDOS) study: A randomized study of orlistat as an adjunct to lifestyle changes for the prevention of type 2 diabetes in obese patients. Diabetes Care. 2004;**27**(1):155-161

[75] Benet LZ, Broccatelli F, Oprea TI. BDDCS applied to over 900 drugs. The AAPS Journal. 2011;**13**(4):519-547

[76] Schoen JC, Erlandson KM, Anderson PL. Clinical pharmacokinetics of antiretroviral drugs in older persons. Expert Opinion on Drug Metabolism & Toxicology. 2013;**9**(5):573-588

[77] Strazielle N, Ghersi-Egea JF. Factors affecting delivery of antiviral drugs to the brain. Reviews in Medical Virology. 2005;**15**(2):105-133

[78] Greenway FL, Fujioka K, Plodkowski RA, Mudaliar S, Guttadauria M, Erickson J, et al. Effect of naltrexone plus bupropion on weight loss in overweight and obese adults (COR-I): A multicentre, randomised, double-blind, placebo-controlled, phase 3 trial. Lancet. 2010;**376**(9741):595-605

[79] Apovian CM, Aronne L, Rubino D, Still C, Wyatt H, Burns C, et al. A randomized, phase 3 trial of naltrexone SR/bupropion SR on weight and obesity-related risk factors (COR-II). Obesity (Silver Spring). 2013;**21**(5):935-943

[80] Wadden TA, Foreyt JP, Foster GD, Hill JO, Klein S, O'Neil PM, et al. Weight loss with naltrexone SR/bupropion SR combination therapy as an adjunct to behavior modification: The COR-BMOD trial. Obesity (Silver Spring). 2011;**19**(1):110-120

[81] Hollander P, Gupta AK, Plodkowski R, Greenway F, Bays H, Burns C, et al. Effects of naltrexone sustained-release/bupropion sustained-release combination therapy on body weight and glycemic parameters in overweight and obese patients

with type 2 diabetes. Diabetes Care. 2013;**36**(12):4022-4029

[82] Yanovski SZ, Yanovski JA. Naltrexone extended-release plus bupropion extended-release for treatment of obesity. Journal of the American Medical Association. 2015;**313**(12):1213-1214

[83] Ornellas T, Chavez B. Naltrexone SR/bupropion SR (Contrave): A new approach to weight loss in obese adults. Pharmacy and Therapeutics. 2011;**36**(5):255-262

[84] Jacobsen LV, Flint A, Olsen AK, Ingwersen SH. Liraglutide in type 2 diabetes mellitus: Clinical pharmacokinetics and pharmacodynamics. Clinical Pharmacokinetics. 2016;**55**(6):657-672

[85] Plum A, Jensen LB, Kristensen JB. In vitro protein binding of liraglutide in human plasma determined by reiterated stepwise equilibrium dialysis. Journal of Pharmaceutical Sciences. 2013;**102**(8):2882-2888

[86] Wadden TA, Hollander P, Klein S, Niswender K, Woo V, Hale PM, et al. Weight maintenance and additional weight loss with liraglutide after low-calorie-diet-induced weight loss: The SCALE maintenance randomized study. International Journal of Obesity. 2013;**37**(11):1443-1451

[87] Croom KF, McCormack PL. Liraglutide: A review of its use in type 2 diabetes mellitus. Drugs. 2009;**69**(14):1985-2004

[88] Malm-Erjefalt M, Ekblom M, Vouis J, Zdravkovic M, Lennernas H. Effect on the gastrointestinal absorption of drugs from different classes in the biopharmaceutics classification system, when treating with liraglutide. Molecular Pharmaceutics. 2015;**12**(11):4166-4173

[89] Wilding JPH, Batterham RL, Calanna S, Davies M, Van Gaal LF, Lingvay I, et al. Once-weekly Semaglutide in adults with overweight or obesity. The New England Journal of Medicine. 2021;**384**(11):989-1002

[90] Jastreboff AM, Aronne LJ, Ahmad NN, Wharton S, Connery L, Alves B, et al. Tirzepatide once weekly for the treatment of obesity. The New England Journal of Medicine. 2022;**387**(3):205-216

[91] Frias JP, Davies MJ, Rosenstock J, Perez Manghi FC, Fernandez Lando L, Bergman BK, et al. Tirzepatide versus Semaglutide once weekly in patients with type 2 diabetes. The New England Journal of Medicine. 2021;**385**(6):503-515

[92] Mallon P. Semaglutide's efficacy in achieving weight loss for those with HIV. Clinicaltrials.gov. 2022 Available from: https://clinicaltrials.gov/ct2/show/NCT04174755

[93] Eckard A. Effects of GLP-l receptor agonists on cardiometabolic alterations in HIV-associated lipohypertrophy. Clinicaltrials.gov; 2022. Available from: https://clinicaltrials.gov/ct2/show/NCT04019197. The AIDS Clinical Trials Group platform is also studying semaglutide effects inPWH (ACTG5371)

[94] Alaber OA, Chandar AK, Dahash BA, Zuzek AC, Rajpal A. 1433-P: Protective effect of GLP-1 receptor agonists (GLP-1 RA) and SGLT2 inhibitors (SGLT2i) against adverse cardiovascular (CV) events in HIV and type 2 diabetes mellitus (T2DM) when compared with metformin alone: A National Database Study. Diabetes. 69(Supplement 1):1433-P DOI: 10.2337/db20-1433-P

[95] Jastreboff AM, Kaplan LM, Frias JP, Wu Q, Du Y, Gurbuz S, et al. Triplehormone-receptor agonist

retatrutide for obesity—A phase 2 trial. The New England Journal of Medicine. 2023;**389**:514-526

[96] Frias JP, Deenadayalan S, Erichsen L, Knop FK, Lingvay I, Macura S, et al. Efficacy and safety of co-administered once-weekly cagrilintide 2.4 mg with once-weekly semaglutide 2.4 mg in type 2 diabetes: A multicentre, randomised, double-blind, active-controlled, phase 2 trial. Lancet. 2023. DOI: 10.1016/S0140-6736(23)01163-7

[97] Apovian CM, McDonnell ME. CagriSema and the link between obesity and type 2 diabetes. Lancet; 2023. S0140-6736(23)01291-6. DOI: 10.1016/S0140-6736(23)01291-6

[98] Wharton S, Blevins T, Connery L, Rosenstock J, Raha S, Liu R, et al. Daily oral GLP-1 receptor agonist Orforglipron for adults with obesity. The New England Journal of Medicine. 2023. DOI: 10.1056/NEJMoa2302392

[99] Cimino C, Binkley A, Swisher R, Short WR. Antiretroviral considerations in HIV-infected patients undergoing bariatric surgery. Journal of Clinical Pharmacy and Therapeutics. 2018;**43**(6):757-767

[100] Alfa-Wali M, Seechurn S, Ayodeji O, Nelson M, Shariq O, Milella M, et al. Outcomes of bariatric surgery in human immunodeficiency virus positive individuals: A single center experience. Minerva Chirurgica. 2016;**71**(4):233-238

[101] Sharma G, Strong AT, Boules M, Tu C, Szomstein S, Rosenthal R, et al. Comparative outcomes of bariatric surgery in patients with and without human immunodeficiency virus. Obesity Surgery. 2018;**28**(4):1070-1079

[102] Paganelli FL, Luyer M, Hazelbag CM, Uh HW, Rogers MRC, Adriaans D, et al. Roux-Y gastric bypass and sleeve gastrectomy directly change gut microbiota composition independent of surgery type. Scientific Reports. 2019;**9**(1):10979

[103] Magouliotis DE, Tasiopoulou VS, Sioka E, Chatedaki C, Zacharoulis D. Impact of bariatric surgery on metabolic and gut microbiota profile: A systematic review and meta-analysis. Obesity Surgery. 2017;**27**(5):1345-1357

[104] Zhang J, Zhang J, Wang R. Gut microbiota modulates drug pharmacokinetics. Drug Metabolism Reviews. 2018;**50**(3):357-368

Section 3

IRIS

Chapter 5

Immune Reconstitution Inflammatory Syndrome and Hodgkin's Lymphoma

Alexander Pivnik and Arsen Vukovich

Abstract

Immune reconstitution inflammatory syndrome (IRIS) is defined as a clinically significant exacerbation of known low-symptomatic serious, more often infectious diseases, in conditions of a significant increase in the level of initially low levels of CD4+ T-lymphocytes in response to highly active antiretroviral therapy (HAART) for HIV infection. Without prior etiotropic therapy for an opportunistic infection, its exacerbation with a pronounced clinical picture during HAART can be fatal for the patient. Lymphomas, including Hodgkin's lymphoma (HL), are considered within the framework of this problem. Unlike other malignant lymphoid tumors that occur with low levels of CD4+ T-lymphocytes, HL develops with elevated levels of CD4+ lymphocytes in response to HAART in HIV-infected patients in the first months of starting antiretroviral treatment. HL was diagnosed in 8% of HIV-infected individuals without HAART. After the appointment of HAART, the frequency of HL increases to 17%. These data allow the problem of IRIS to be considered as the main one in the study of the etiology and pathogenesis of HL in HIV-infected patients.

Keywords: IRIS, Hodgkin lymphoma, HAART, aggressive lymphoma, hematology

1. Introduction

Classical HL is a monoclonal tumor, the substrate of which is Reed-Sternberg cells (R-SH) and Hodgkin cells, which originate from the germinal center of the follicles. After, it was introduced into the clinical practice of HAART the incidence of aggressive lymphomas and Kaposi's angiosarcoma decreased many times, and the incidence of HL, on the contrary, increased to 17% [1]. We are going to introduce our study of HL and IRIS.

2. Hodgkin's lymphoma: definition, history, and diagnostics

Hodgkin's lymphoma (HL; Hodgkin's disease, lymphogranulomatosis) is a disease that includes classical HL and nodular lymphocyte-predominant Hodgkin lymphoma (NLPHL). Classical HL is a monoclonal tumor, the substrate of which is

Reed-Sternberg cells (R-SH) and Hodgkin cells, which originate from the B cells of the germinal center of the follicles. They make up about 1% of the total mass of tumor tissue, which consists of reactive, non-tumor T- and B- lymphocytes with an admixture of granulocytes and macrophages. Histological variants of HL were determined: lymphoid predominance, mixed-cell variant, nodular sclerosis, and lymphoid depletion. Later, the nodular variant is divided into two: the first type and the second type. In the first type, a small number of R-SH cells are distributed and scattered in the histological specimen. The prognosis of the disease is favorable. In the second type of variant with nodular sclerosis, tumor cells form syncytium. The prognosis is unfavorable. Hypereosinophilia in the specimen also indicates an unfavorable prognosis.

Hodgkin's lymphoma was first described in six patients in 1832 by Thomas Hodgkin as "a disease in which the lymph nodes and spleen are affected." After 23 years, S. Wilkes called this condition "Hodgkin's disease", having studied the observations described by T. Hodgkin and added 11 of his own to them [2]. The term "lymphogranulomatosis" was introduced in 1904, at the VII Congress of German Pathologists in Vienna, and for a long time, the process was differentiated with tuberculosis. In 1971, at the Ann Arbor conference, a classification was adopted for the staging of lymphomas from I to IV with the presence of clinical symptoms of intoxication (B) and without them (A). In 1988, Costwolds adopted additions: a massive tumor (bulky) X and a letter representation of the affected organs (S – spleen, H – hepar, etc.) [3]. In the classification of tumors of hematopoietic and lymphoid tissues, WHO 2001 approved the name "Hodgkin's lymphoma". Later, a nodular lymphocyte-predominant Hodgkin lymphoma (NLPHL) was isolated in which the addition of rituximab to the regimens of chemotherapy is required, which may differ from those developed for HL [4]. During immunohistochemical examination, the basic markers of HL were identified: CD30, CD25, and CD15. Up to 70% of patients are carriers of the Epstein-Barr virus (EBV). The problem of EBV oncogenesis in lymphomas is being intensively studied, but it has not yet been solved [5]. The generally accepted treatment regimens for HL are ABVD AVD, BEACOP-14, BEACOPP-escalated, DHAP, and ESHAP. In some patients, autologous hematopoietic stem cell transplantation is used at the stage of consolidation after high-dose chemotherapy, more often with relapses/refractory course of the tumor.

Before starting chemotherapy, young men are offered cryopreservation of sperm, and women are offered cryopreservation of follicles.

According to the staging system adopted in Ann Arbor [6], bone marrow involvement qualifies as stage IV of tumor spread. However, the bone marrow naturally belongs to the hematopoiesis system, and the stage should be designated as III (personal point of view of the authors). Bone marrow damage is not a risk factor. Trepanobiopsy is not performed during the initial diagnosis of HL, but in case of relapse, this procedure is mandatory. Bone marrow involvement in primary HL patients according to bilateral trepanobiopsy is confirmed only in 12–14% of cases [1, 7]. According to the results of PET-CT, bone marrow involvement is registered much more often in 54% of patients [8].

3. Immune reconstitution inflammatory syndrome

The first reports on the side effects of HAART appeared in 1997. As the viral load decreased and the CD4+ T-lymphocyte count in the blood increased, reflecting the effectiveness of antiretroviral treatment for HIV. In the past few years, the effectiveness of antiretroviral treatment for HIV infection has led to a resurgence of known, previously asymptomatic diseases. For example, these include pulmonary and extrapulmonary forms of tuberculosis, including atypical nontuberculous mycobacterioses: paratuberculosis, leprosy, fungal infections, parasitosis, contagious mollusks, cryptococcal infection, toxoplasmosis, shingles, leishmaniasis, and exacerbation of syphilis with a return of the initial clinical picture [9–19]. In addition, Guillain-Barré syndrome has been described in patients with HIV infection on HAART [20]. A. Weetman reports thyroiditis occurring 15 months after starting HAART [21].

In 2000, the Annals of Internal Medicine journal J.A. DeSimone et al. first described a new syndrome [22]. It is based on the phenomenon called IRIS (Immune Reconstitution Inflammatory Syndrome). In Russian literature, IRIS is recognized to be an inflammatory immune reaction.

The most frequent description of IRIS is tuberculosis-associated. There are several criteria and three categories of coinfection [23–30].

IRIS and tuberculosis occur in almost 1/3 of all HIV-infected patients on HAART [31, 32]. There is an urgent need of tuberculosis therapy prior to the administration of HAART [32, 33].

C.C. Chang et al. concluded that low levels of CD4+ T- lymphocytes and protein in the spinal fluid increase the risk of death in cryptococcal meningitis [34]. I. Sereti points out that HAART should be administered only after microbiological confirmation of cerebrospinal fluid sterility [35]. Cryptococcal meningitis is detected within 2 weeks to 4 months from the start of HAART [36–38].

Uveitis after initiating HAART is recognized as IRU (Immune Reconstitution Uveitis) and is found in 37.5% of cases [39]. HAART reduced the number of cases of CMV retinitis by 90%. Without HAART, uveitis occurred at CD4+ T-lymphocyte levels of 50 cells/μL or lower, and with HAART, it occurred at 200 cells/μL or higher [40–44].

Literature in the Russian language provides the first mention of IRIS in work of N.V. Matievskaya in 2012. The author described 73 patients with HIV infection, indicating the occurrence of severe IRIS in eight of them. The patients were diagnosed with purulent meningitis, toxoplasmosis, tuberculosis, and lymphomas, including HL in one patient. Manifestations of IRIS were noted after 1 week and up to 1 year from the start of HAART. HL was diagnosed 1 year after the start of antiretroviral therapy. Lethal outcomes occurred in five patients [45].

Panteleev A.M. reports on corticosteroid treatment in IRIS and tuberculosis [46]. A.M. Bitneva et al. reports the results of data analysis of 179 patients observed in a phthisiology department, 21 of which with IRIS [47]. The Belarusian authors Tyushchenko T.V. and Tsyrkunov V.M. reported that 47 patients with HIV infection died of opportunistic infections 3 months after the initiation of HAART [48]. I.M. Ulyukin notes the importance of careful monitoring in patients taking HAART with previous tuberculosis background [49].

IRIS also occurs in patients without HIV infection after treatment of tumor and autoimmune diseases with immunosuppressants and corticosteroid hormones [50].

IRIS has been described by P. Vishnu et al. in three patients with Burkitt's lymphoma (BL) diagnosed 20–24 weeks after HAART initiation, with CD4+ T-lymphocytes at 323, 553 and 293 cells/μL, respectively. In two patients, the viral load was not determined. Of the patients examined, one patient died, and two others achieved complete remission. The authors in their literature review of 2000–2013 found descriptions of only three patients with LB diagnosed 8–28 weeks after initiation of HAART. Lymphoma was diagnosed at an average CD4+ T- lymphocyte count of 277 cells/μL. Two patients died from the progression of LB, and one achieved complete remission [51].

Although HL is not an HIV-indicating malignancy, the incidence of this particular malignant lymphoid tumor is about 10 times higher in HIV-positive populations than in HIV-negative ones [52]. Despite the fact that the incidence of many opportunistic infections is decreasing in the "HAART era" [53, 54] incidence of HL in HIV-infected patients is increasing [55–60].

The largest number of patients with HIV infection and HL were described by R.J. Biggar et al. in 2006. Authors analyzed 317,428 cases of HIV infection of which classical HL was diagnosed in 173 cases. The mixed-cell variant was predominant (54%). It was shown that the risk of LC in HIV-infected patients with a CD4+ T-lymphocyte count of 225–249 cells/μL increases 10-fold compared to the general population. The authors also confirmed that the mixed-cell variant of HL with frequent detection of Epstein-Barr virus prevailed [56].

A multicenter study in which the authors linked the development of HL in HIV-infected patients with IRIS analyzed data of 64,368 HIV-infected patients from 1992 to 2009 in France, of whom 187 developed HL. This study did not specify what level of CD4+ T- lymphocytes prior to the development of HL. More than half of these patients were diagnosed with HL within the first 3 months of HAART initiation. An important conclusion is that the risk of HL diagnosis in patients who received HAART is generally low. However, it is shown that patients with a CD4+ T-lymphocyte level of at least 500 cells/μL have an almost 10-fold increased risk of HL compared to patients with a CD4+ T-lymphocyte level of 50–99 cells/μL [59].

J. Bohlius et al. indicate that a decreased level of CD4+ T-lymphocytes in patients receiving HAART correlates with an increased risk of developing HL [61]. A. Kowalkowski et al. reported the results of a multicenter analysis of 31,056 patients with HIV infection from 1985 to 2010 in Houston, of whom 196 had HL. It was shown that in patients with HL, CD4+ T-lymphocyte levels continued to decline 3–6 months after initiation of HAART. After 3 years of follow-up, it was found that the risk of developing HL in patients who received HAART doubled during the first year. It is noted that patients with CD4+ T-lymphocytes level of 200–350 cells/μL are in the group with the highest risk of HL [62]. Long-term HAART has been shown to reduce the risk of developing HL. Thus, HL was diagnosed in 211 of 31,576 patients with HIV infection who received HAART [63]. D. Gotti et al. report on 5087 HIV-infected patients followed up for 10 years, of whom 30 patients developed HL. It was shown that the risk of HL increases within 6 months of starting HAART [64]. Increased incidence of HL in HIV-infected patients receiving HAART has also been reported in other studies [65, 66].

Thus, in the literature, there are reports of better results of antitumor therapy in combination with HAART in patients with multiple myeloma and concomitant HIV infection than in the group without HIV infection [67].

4. Our study

4.1 Materials and methods

From 2002 to 2019, we observed 85 patients with HIV infection, HL, and concomitant hepatitis C and/or B. For technical reasons, data for 2008–2011 were excluded from the analysis. Thus, the study included 85 patients aged 20–74 years (median 35 years), 67% male.

4.2 Results

Immunohistochemical study of tumor biopsy specimens revealed that 60 (70%) patients were EBV-positive. Coinfection with hepatitis C and B viruses was detected in 81 (95%) patients with HL. The level of CD4+ lymphocytes before the start of anti-cancer treatment for HL was about 400/mcL, and the viral load was above 100,000 copies/mcL. Before the start of chemotherapy, seven patients died. These patients presented with stage IVB HL, massive tumor lesions, and B-symptoms and died from tumor progression and opportunistic infections.

The treatment was carried out according to internationally accepted chemo-therapy regimens: 6 courses of ABVD, 6 courses of BEACOPP-14, and 6 courses of BEACOPP-escalated with or without subsequent radiation therapy. Without exception, all patients underwent HAART simultaneously with anticancer treatment. In cases of a combination of HL, HIV infection and hepatitis B and/or C, simultaneous treatment of all three diseases is carried out. In the case of hepatitis C, direct-acting drugs orally are used for 12 weeks, with complete eradication of the virus achieved in 96% of cases. After the end of chemotherapy treatment of HL, the level of CD4+ lymphocytes increased to 700/μl, and the viral load decreased significantly to undetectable at the sensitivity threshold of the method of 25 copies/μl and below. It should be emphasized that over the entire historical period of observation under conditions of strict monitoring from 2002 to 2019, we did not observe relapses of HL. And as a consequence, we have not had to refer patients for transplantation of autologous hematopoietic stem cells. At the time of writing the article, 70 patients remained in complete remission of HL, confirmed by CT or PET-CT. See **Table 1**.

Index	**Number, n (%)**
Total number of patients	85 (100)
Sex	
Men	58 (69)
Women	27 (31)
Median (range) age, years	35 (20–74)
HL variant	
Lymphoid predominance	4 (4.5)
Mixed cell	68 (80)
nodular sclerosis	5 (6)
lymphoid depletion	8 (9.5)
HL stage by Ann Arbor	
I	0 (0)
II	17 (20)
III	17 (20)
IV	51 (60)
HIV infection	
The level of CD4+ lymphocytes at the diagnosis of HL, cells/μl	
> 500	51 (60)

Index	Number, n (%)
500–350	17 (20)
200–350	10 (12)
< 200	7 (8)
Viral load, copies/μl	
<10,000	22 (26)
10,000–50,000	34 (40)
50,000–100,000	17 (20)
>100,000	12 (14)
Viral hepatitis	
Only C	60 (70)
Only B	9 (11)
Combination of C and B	12 (14)
Anticancer treatment regimen	
ABVD	60 (70)
BEACOPP-escalated	10 (12)
BEACOPP-14	7 (8)
Another	8 (10)
EBV infection	
Positive	60 (70)
Negative	25 (30)
Treatment results	
Remission	70 (82)
Complete remission	60 (86)
Partial remission	0 (0)
Stabilization	10 (14)
Progression	0 (0)
Relapses/refractory course	0 (0)
Mortality	
Before starting PCT	7 (8)
From complications of PCT	8 (10)

Table 1.
Clinical characteristics of patients.

5. Conclusions

The pathogenesis of IRIS is unclear. Obviously, an increased number of CD4+ T-lymphocytes plays an important role in the pathogenesis of IRIS. In addition, elevated levels of cytokines such as interferon-γ, interleukin-6, and tumor necrosis factor α can be detected, simultaneously [68–77]. Risk factors for the development of IRIS include increased levels of T- lymphocytes, CD4+, CD4+ to CD8+ T-lymphocyte ratio, the drop in the viral load after 90 days of HAART, and its early administration in case of opportunistic infections. When risk factors were taken into account, the decrease in viral load was significant, and the baseline CD4+ T-lymphocyte level was about 200 cl/μL [78, 79].

The incidence of HL in the "HAART era" has increased markedly [80, 81]. An essential feature of HL is the microenvironment of reactive cells in the tumor mass. Neoplastic-Reed-Sternberg cells and Hodgkin's cells usually make up 0.1–1% among the tumor microenvironment cells [82, 83]. However, tumor cells actively produce cytokines and chemokines, providing influx of activated CD4+ T- lymphocytes, as well as cells expressing CD40, CD26, histiocytes, and other cellular elements.

Thus, the experience of foreign and domestic researchers allows us to consider IRIS as one of the main problems in the study of the etiology and pathogenesis of HL in HIV-infected patients. The specificity of the directed action of T cells to the tumor antigens, which have not yet been elucidated, remains open. In this connection, it is strongly recommended to continue research in this direction.

Generalization of our own data allows us to conclude that HL in patients with HIV infection with standard chemotherapy regimens with simultaneous HAART gives better results in comparison with the HL group without HIV infection. These results are consistent with the reports available for another malignant lymphatic tumor. Thus, there are reports in the literature about better results of antitumor therapy in combination with HAART in patients with multiple myeloma and concomitant HIV infection than in the group without HIV infection [84].

Based on our own 17-year clinical experience in treating patients with HIV and HIV infection (antitumor treatment and HAART), we allowed ourselves to express a seditious idea about the possible use of HAART in hematological malignant tumors without concomitant HIV infection, although this requires serious research and evidence.

Deciphering the etiology and pathogenesis of HL is most likely possible when solving the IRIS problem and clarifying the issues of EBV oncogenesis.

Bone marrow involvement in primary patients with HL does not serve as an unfavorable prognostic sign and does not require histological confirmation based on the results of a trepanobiopsy study. At the same time, with relapses of HL, trepanobiopsy is a mandatory diagnostic procedure since the involvement of bone marrow in relapses is regarded as an extremely unfavorable prognostic factor. Cryopreservation of sperm and storage of follicles in persons of reproductive age is desirable.

A clear knowledge of the specificity and sensitivity of the T-cell reaction in the formation of granulomas is needed. The unraveling of this phenomenon may shed light on the possible deciphering of the pathogenetic mechanisms of the occurrence and development of HL in the general population without HIV infection.

Author details

Alexander Pivnik and Arsen Vukovich*
Peoples' Friendship University of Russia, Russia, Moscow

*Address all correspondence to: arsen.vukovic@gmail.com

References

[1] Breen RA, Smith CJ, Bettinson H, et al. Paradoxical reactions during tuberculosis treatment in patients with and without HIV co-infection. Thorax. 2004;**59**(8):704-707. DOI: 10.1136/thx.2003.019224

[2] Geller SA. Comments on the anniversary of the description of Hodgkin's disease. Journal of the National Medical Association. 1984;**76**(8):815-817

[3] Lister TA, Crowther D, Sutcliffe SB, et al. Report of a committee convened to discuss the evaluation and staging of patients with Hodgkin's disease: Cotswold's meeting. Journal of Clinical Oncology. 1989;7(11):1630-1636. DOI: 10.1200/jco.1989.7.11.1630

[4] Demina EA, Tumyan GS, Chekan AA, et al. Rare disease – Nodular lymphocyte-predominant Hodgkin's lymphoma: Literature review and own data. Clinical Onkogematology. 2014;7(4):522-532

[5] Gurtsevich VE. Epstein-Barr virus and classical Hodgkin's lymphoma. Clinical Oncohematology. 2016;**9**(2):101-114. DOI: 10.21320/2500-2139-2016-9-2-101-114. In Russian

[6] Carbone PP, Kaplan HS, Musshoff K, et al. Report of the Committee on Hodgkin's Disease Staging Classification. Cancer Res. Nov 1971;**31**(11):1860-1861. PMID: 5121694

[7] Rasstrigin NA. Alternating polychemotherapy of lymphog-ranulomatosis: Dis. cand. RAMS. Sciences. 1999:124

[8] Aslanidi IP, Mukhortova OV, Katunina TA, et al. Positron emission tomography in modern management of lymphomas. Clinical Oncohematology. 2015;**8**(1):13-25. DOI: 10.21320/2500-2139-2015-8-1-13-25

[9] Lai RP, Meintjes G, Wilkinson RJ. HIV-1 tuberculosis-associated immune reconstitution inflammatory syndrome. Seminars in Immunopathology. 2016;**38**(2):185-198. DOI: 10.1007/s00281-015-0532-2

[10] Richter E, Wessling J, Lugering N, et al. Mycobacterium avium subsp. paratuberculosis infection in a patient with HIV, Germany. Emerging Infectious Diseases. 2002;**8**(7):729-731. DOI: 10.3201/eid0807.010388

[11] Amerson EH, Maurer TA. Immune reconstitution inflammatory syndrome and tropical dermatoses. Dermatologic Clinics. 2011;**29**(1):39-43. DOI: 10.1016/j.det.2010.09.007

[12] Gupta A, Sharma YK, Ghogre M, et al. Giant molluscum contagiosum unmasked probably during an immune reconstitution inflammatory syndrome. Indian Journal of Sexually Transmitted Diseases and AIDS. 2018;**39**(2):139-140. DOI: 10.4103/ijstd.IJSTD_60_16

[13] Balasko A, Keynan Y. Shedding light on IRIS: From pathophysiology to treatment of cryptococcal meningitis and immune reconstitution inflammatory syndrome in HIV-infected individuals. HIV Medicine. 2019;**20**(1):1-10. DOI: 10.1111/hiv.12676

[14] Martin-Blondel G, Alvarez M, Delobel PV, et al. Toxoplasmic encephalitis IRIS in HIV-infected patients: A case series and review of the literature. Journal of Neurology, Neurosurgery, and Psychiatry. 2010;**82**(6):691-693. DOI: 10.1136/jnnp.2009.199919

[15] Karavellas MP, Lowder CY, Macdonald C, et al. Immune recovery vitritis associated with inactive cytomegalovirus retinitis: A new syndrome. Archives of Ophthalmology. 1998;**116**(2):169-175. DOI: 10.1001/archopht.116.2.169

[16] Boulougoura A, Sereti I. HIV infection and immune activation: The role of coinfections. Current Opinion in HIV and AIDS. 2016;**11**(2):191-200. DOI: 10.1097/COH.0000000000000241

[17] Hosoda T, Uehara Y, Kasuga K, et al. An HIV-infected patient with acute retinal necrosis as immune reconstitution inflammatory syndrome due to varicellazoster virus. AIDS. 2020;**34**(5):795-796. DOI: 10.1097/QAD.0000000000002477

[18] Auyeung P, French MA, Hollingsworth PN. Immune restoration disease associated with leishmania donovani infection following antiretroviral therapy for HIV infection. Journal of Microbiology, Immunology, and Infection. 2010;**43**(1):74-76. DOI: 10.1016/S1684-1182(10)60011-4

[19] Alcedo S, Newby R, Montenegro J, et al. Immune reconstitution inflammatory syndrome associated with secondary syphilis: Dermatologic, neurologic and ophthalmologic compromise in an HIV patient. International Journal of STD & AIDS. 2019;**30**(5):509-511. DOI: 10.1177/0956462418813045

[20] Mathukumalli NL, Ali N, Kanikannan MA, Yareeda S. Worsening GuillainBarre syndrome: harbinger of IRIS in HIV? BMJ Case Reports. 2017;**2017**:221874. DOI: 10.1136/bcr-2017-221874

[21] Weetman A. Immune reconstitution syndrome and the thyroid. Best Practice & Research Clinical Endocrinology & Metabolism. 2009;**23**(6):693-702. DOI: 10.1 016/j. beem.2009.07.003

[22] DeSimone JA, Pomerantz RJ, Babinchak TJ. Inflammatory reactions in HIV1-infected persons after initiation of highly active antiretroviral therapy. Annals of Internal Medicine. 2000;**133**(6):447-454. DOI: 10.7326/0003-4819-133-6-200009190-00013

[23] Meintjes G, Lawn SD, Scano F, et al. Tuberculosis-associated immune reconstitution inflammatory syndrome: Case definitions for use in resource-limited settings. The Lancet Infectious Diseases. 2008;**8**(8):516-523. DOI: 10.1016/s1473-3099(08)70184-1

[24] Shelburne SA, Montes M, Hamill RJ. Immune reconstitution inflammatory syndrome: More answers, more questions. The Journal of Antimicrobial Chemotherapy. 2005;**57**(2):167-170. DOI: 10.1093/jac/dki444

[25] French MA, Price P, Stone SF. Immune restoration disease after antiretroviral therapy. AIDS. 2004;**18**(12):1615-1627. DOI: 10.1097/01.aids.0000131375.21070.06

[26] Lai RPJ, Nakiwala JK, Meintjes G, Wilkinson RJ. The immunopathogenesis of the HIV tuberculosis immune reconstitution inflammatory syndrome. European Journal of Immunology. 2013;**43**(8):1995-2002. DOI: 10.1002/eji.201343632

[27] WHO. Improving the diagnosis and treatment of smear-negative pulmonary and extrapulmonary tuberculosis among adults and adolescents: Recommendations for HIV-prevalent and resource-constrained settings. In: Stop TB Department, Department of HIV/AIDS. Geneva, Switzerland: World Health Organization; 2006

[28] Manosuthi W, Kiertiburanakul S, Phoorisri T, Sungkanuparph S. Immune reconstitution inflammatory syndrome of tuberculosis among HIV-infected patients receiving antituberculous and antiretroviral therapy. The Journal of Infection. 2006;**53**(6):357-363. DOI: 10.1016/j.jinf.2006.01.002

[29] Lawn SD, Myer L, Bekker LG, Wood R. Tuberculosis-associated immune reconstitution disease: Incidence, risk factors and impact in an antiretroviral treatment service in South Africa. Acquired Immunodeficiency Syndrome. 2007;**21**(3):335-341. DOI: 10.1097/QAD.0b013e328011efac

[30] Narita M, Ashkin D, Hollender ES, Pitchenik AE. Paradoxical worsening of tuberculosis following antiretroviral therapy in patients with AIDS. American Journal of Respiratory and Critical Care Medicine. 1998;**158**(1):157-161. DOI: 10.1164/ajrccm.158.1.9712001

[31] Breton G, Duval X, Estellat C, et al. Determinants of immune reconstitution inflammatory syndrome in HIV type 1-infected patients with tuberculosis after initiation of antiretroviral therapy. Clinical Infectious Diseases. 2004;**39**(11):1709-1712. DOI: 10.1086/425742

[32] Meintjes G, Wilkinson RJ, Morroni C, et al. Randomized placebo-controlled trial of prednisone for paradoxical tuberculosis-associated immune reconstitution inflammatory syndrome. Acquired Immunodeficiency Syndrome. 2010;**24**(15):2381-2390. DOI: 10.1097/QAD.0b013e32833dfc68

[33] Michailidis C, Pozniak AL, Mandalia S, et al. Clinical characteristics of IRIS syndrome in patients with HIV and tuberculosis. Antiviral Therapy. 2005;**10**(3):417-422

[34] Chang CC, Dorasamy AA, Gosnell BI, et al. Clinical and mycological predictors of cryptococcosis-associated immune reconstitution inflammatory syndrome. Acquired Immunodeficiency Syndrome. 2013;**27**(13):2089-2099. DOI: 10.1097/qad.0b013e3283614a8d

[35] Sereti I. Immune reconstruction inflammatory syndrome in HIV infection: Beyond what meets the eye. Archive of Topics in Antiviral Medicine. 2020;**27**(4):106-111

[36] Jenny-Avital ER, Abadi M. Immune reconstitution cryptococcosis after initiation of successful highly active antiretroviral therapy. Clinical Infectious Diseases. 2002;**35**(12):128-133. DOI: 10.1086/344467

[37] Somnuek S, Scott GF, Ploenchan C, et al. Cryptococcal immune reconstitution inflammatory syndrome after antiretroviral therapy in AIDS patients with cryptococcal meningitis: A prospective Multicenter study. Clinical Infectious Diseases. 2009;**6**(15):931-934. DOI: 10.1086/605497

[38] Meya DB, Okurut S, Zziwa G, et al. HIV-associated cryptococcal ImmuneReconstitution inflammatory syndrome is associated with aberrant T cell function and increased cytokine responses. Journal of Fungi. 2019;**5**(2):42. DOI: 10.3390/jof5020042

[39] Arevalo JF, Mendoza AJ, FerrettiI Y. Immune recovery uveitis In AIDS Patients with cytomegalovirus retinitis treated with highly active antiretroviral therapy In Venezuela. Retina. 2003;**23**(4):495-502. DOI: 10.1097/00006982-200308000-00009

[40] Jabs DA. Cytomegalovirus retinitis and the acquired immunodeficiency syndrome-bench to bedside: LXVII Edward Jackson memorial lecture. American Journal of Ophthalmology. 2011;**151**(2):198-216. DOI: 10.1016/j.ajo.2010.10.018

[41] Kaplan JE, Benson C, Holmes KK, et al. Centers for Disease Control and Prevention (CDC). Guidelines for prevention and treatment of opportunistic infections in HIV-infected adults and adolescents: recommendations from CDC, the National Institutes of Health, and the HIV Medicine Association of the Infectious Diseases Society of America, National Institutes of Health, HIV Medicine Association of the Infectious Diseases Society of America. MMWR Recommendations and Reports. 2009;**58**(RR-4):1-207. DOI: 10.1037/e537722009-001

[42] Jacobson MA, Zegans M, Pavan P. Cytomegalovirus retinitis after initiation of highly active antiretroviral therapy. Lancet. 1997;**349**(9063):1443-1445. DOI: 10.1016/ s0140-6736(96)11431-8

[43] Mitchell SM, Membrey WL, Youle MS, et al. Cytomegalovirus retinitis after the initiation of highly active antiretroviral therapy: A 2-year prospective study. The British Journal of Ophthalmology. 1999;**83**(6):652-655. DOI: 10.1136/bjo.83.6.652

[44] Jabs DA, Ahuja A, Van Natta M, et al. Course of cytomegalovirus retinitis in the era of highly active antiretroviral therapy: Five-year outcomes. Ophthalmology. 2010;**117**(11):2152-2161.e2. DOI: 10.1016/j.ophtha.2010.03.031

[45] Matievskaya NV. Immune reconstitution inflammatory syndrome: Risk factors, clinical manifestations, outcomes, prevention. Vestnik Baltiiskogo Federal'nogo Universiteta im. I. Kanta. 2012;7:44-51

[46] Panteleev AM. Patogenez, klinika, diagnostika i lechenie tuberkuleza u bol'nykh VICh-infektsiei. (pathogenesis, clinical features, diagnosis, and treatment of tuberculosis in patients with HIV infection). [dissertation]. Saint Petersburg. 2012:236

[47] Bitneva AM, Kozlova TP, Savintseva EV. Characteristics of the start and course of immune reconstitution inflammatory syndrome in pulmonary tuberculosis. Problemy Nauki. 2017;**6**(19):104-105

[48] Tishchenko TV, Tsyrkunov VM. Immune reconstitution inflammatory syndrome in HIV-positive patients: Clinicopathological aspects. Zdravookhranenie (Minsk). 2017;**10**:5-11

[49] Ulyukin IM. HIV-infection: Characteristics of immune reconstitution on specific therapy of tuberculosis. Klinicheskaya Patofiziologiya. 2017;**23**(2):29-33

[50] Sun H-Y, Singh N. Immune reconstitution inflammatory syndrome in nonHIV immunocompromised patients. Current Opinion in Infectious Diseases. 2009;**22**(4):394-402. DOI: 10.1097/QCO.0b013e32832d7aff

[51] Vishnu P, Dorer RP, Aboulafia DM. Immune reconstitution inflammatory syndrome-associated Burkitt lymphoma after combination antiretroviral therapy in HIV-infected patients. Clinical Lymphoma, Myeloma and Leukemia. 2015;**15**(1):23-29. DOI: 10.1016/j.clml.2014.09.009

[52] Serraino D, Boschini A, Carrieri P, et al. Cancer risk among men with, or at risk of, HIV infection in southern Europe. Acquired Immunodeficiency Syndrome. 2000;**14**(5):553-559. DOI: 10.1097/00002030-200003310-00011

[53] Noy A. Update on HIV lymphoma. Current Oncology Reports. 2007;**9**(5):384-390. DOI: 10.1007/s11912-007-0052-x

[54] Franceschi S, Dal Maso L, Pezzotti P, et al. Incidence of AIDS-defining cancers

after AIDS diagnosis among people with AIDS in Italy, 1986-1998. Journal of Acquired Immune Deficiency Syndromes. 2003;**34**(1):84-90. DOI:10.1097/00126334-200309010-00013

[55] Carbone A, Gloghini A, Larocca LM, et al. Human immunodeficiency virus associated Hodgkin's disease derives from post-germinal center B cells. Blood. 1999;**93**(7):2319-2326. DOI: 10.1182/blood.V93.7.2319

[56] Biggar RJ, Jaffe ES, Goedert JJ, et al. Hodgkin lymphoma and immunodeficiency in persons with HIV/AIDS. Blood. 2006;**108**(12):3786-3791. DOI: 10.1182/blood-2006-05-024109

[57] Engels EA, Pfeiffer RM, Goedert JJ, et al. Trends in cancer risk among people with AIDS in the United States 1980-2002. Journal of Acquired Immune Deficiency Syndromes. 2006;**20**(12):1645-1654. DOI: 10.1097/01.aids.0000238411.75324.59

[58] Dauby N, De Wit S, Delforge M, et al. Characteristics of non-AIDS-defining malignancies in the HAART era: A clinico-epidemiological study. Journal of the International AIDS Society. 2011;**14**(1):16. DOI: 10.1186/1758-2652-14-16

[59] Stein H, Mann R, Delsol G, et al. Hodgkin lymphoma. In: Jaffe ES, Harris NL, Stein H, Vardiman JW, editors. World Health Organization Classification of Tumors: Pathology and Genetics of Tumors of Haematopoietic and Lymphoid Tissues. Lyon: IARC Press; 2001. pp. 237-252

[60] Lanoy E, Rosenberg PS, Fily F, et al. HIV-associated Hodgkin lymphoma during the first months on combination antiretroviral therapy. Blood. 2011;**118**(1):44-49. DOI: 10.1182/blood-2011-02-339275

[61] Bohlius J, Schmidlin K, Boue F, et al. Collaboration of observational HIV epidemiological research Europe. HIV-1-related Hodgkin lymphoma in the era of combination antiretroviral therapy: Incidence and evolution of CD4+ T-cell lymphocytes. Blood. 2011;**117**(23):6100-6108. DOI: 10.1182/blood-2010-08-301531

[62] Kowalkowski MA, Mims MP, Amiran ES, et al. Effect of immune reconstitution on the incidence of HIV-related Hodgkin lymphoma. PLoS One. 2013;**8**(10):e77409. DOI: 10.1371/journal.pone.0077409

[63] Kowalkowski MA, Mims MA, Day RS, et al. Longer duration of combination antiretroviral therapy reduces the risk of Hodgkin lymphoma: A cohort study of HIV-infected male veterans. Cancer Epidemiology. 2014;**38**(4):386-392. DOI: 10.1016/j. canep.2014.05.009

[64] Gotti D, Danesi M, Calabresi A, et al. Clinical characteristics, incidence, and risk factors of HIV-related Hodgkin lymphoma in the era of combination antiretroviral therapy. AIDS Patient Care and STDs. 2013;**27**(5):259. DOI: 10.1089/apc.2012.0424

[65] Patel P, Hanson DL, Sullivan PS, et al. Incidence of types of cancer among HIV-infected persons compared with the general population in the United States, 1992-2003. Annals of Internal Medicine. 2008;**148**(10):728-736. DOI: 10.7326/0003-4819-148-.10-200805200-00005

[66] Yotsumoto M, Hagiwara S, Ajisawa A, et al. Clinical characteristics of human immunodeficiency virus-associated Hodgkin lymphoma patients in Japan. International Journal of Hematology. 2012;**96**(2):247-253. DOI: 10.1007/s12185-012-1127-5

[67] Pivnik AV, Tumanova MV, Seregin NV. Lymphomas in

HIV-infected patients: A review of the literature. Clinical Oncohematology. 2014;7(3):264-277

[68] Sombogaard F, Franssen EJF, Terpstra WE. Outcome effects of antiretroviral drug combinations in HIV-positive patients with chemotherapy for lymphoma: A retrospective analysis. International Journal of Clinical Pharmacy. 2018;**40**(5):1402-1408. DOI: 10.1007/s11096-018-0620-1

[69] Eschke M, Piehler D, Schulze B, et al. A novel experimental model of Cryptococcus neoformans-related immune reconstitution inflammatory syndrome (IRIS) provides insights into pathogenesis. European Journal of Immunology. 2015;**45**(12):333950. DOI: 10.1002/eji.201545689

[70] Tadokera R, Wilkinson KA, Meintjes GA, et al. Role of the interleukin 10 family of cytokines in patients with immune reconstitution inflammatory syndrome associated with HIV infection and tuberculosis. The Journal of Infectious Diseases. 2013;**207**(7):1148-1156. DOI: 10.1093/infdis/jit002

[71] Sereti I, Rodger AJ, French MA. Biomarkers in immune reconstitution inflammatory syndrome: Signals from pathogenesis. Current Opinion in HIV and AIDS. 2010;**5**(6):504-510. DOI: 10.1097/COH.0b013e32833ed774

[72] Chang CC, Lim A, Omarjee S, et al. Cryptococcosis-IRIS is associated with lower cryptococcus-specific IFN-γ responses before antiretroviral therapy but not higher T-cell responses during therapy. The Journal of Infectious Diseases. 2013;**208**(6):898-906. DOI: 10.1093/infdis/jit271

[73] Meya DB, Manabe YC, Boulware DR, Janoff EN. The immunopathogenesis of cryptococcal immune reconstitution inflammatory syndrome: Understanding a conundrum. Current Opinion in Infectious Diseases. 2016;**29**(1):10-22. DOI: 10.1097/QCO.0000000000000224

[74] de Sa NBR, Ribeiro-Alves M, da Silva TP, et al. Clinical and genetic markers associated with tuberculosis, HIV-1 infection, and TB/HIV-immune reconstitution inflammatory syndrome outcomes. BMC Infectious Diseases. 2020;**20**(1):59. DOI: 10.1186/s12879-020-4786-5

[75] Crane M, Matthews G, Lewin SR. Hepatitis virus immune restoration disease of the liver. Current Opinion in HIV and AIDS. 2008;**3**(4):446-452. DOI: 10.1097/ coh.0b013e3282fdc953

[76] Ravimohan S, Tamuhla N, Nfanyana K, et al. Robust reconstitution of tuberculosis-specific polyfunctional CD4+ T-cell responses and rising systemic interleukin 6 in paradoxical tuberculosis-associated immune reconstitution inflammatory syndrome. Clinical Infectious Diseases. 2016;**62**(6):795-803. DOI: 10.1093/cid/ civ978

[77] Stek C, Allwood B, Du Bruyn E, et al. The effect of HIV-associated tuberculosis, tuberculosis-IRIS and prednisone on lung function. The European Respiratory Journal. 2020;**55**(3):1901692. DOI: 10.1183/13993003.01692-2019

[78] Dhasmana DJ, Dheda K, Ravn P, et al. Immune reconstitution inflammatory syndrome in HIV-infected patients receiving antiretroviral therapy: Pathogenesis, clinical manifestations and management. Drugs. 2008;**68**:191-208. DOI:10.2165/00003495-200868020-00004

[79] Beishuizen SJ, Geerlings SE. Immune reconstitution inflammatory syndrome: Immunopathogenesis, risk factors, diagnosis and prevention. The Netherlands Journal of Medicine. 2009;**67**(10):327-331

[80] Herida A, Mary-Krause M, Kaphan R, et al. Incidence of non AIDS-defining cancers before and during the highly active antiretroviral therapy era in a cohort of human immunodeficiency virus-infected patients. Journal of Clinical Oncology. 2003;**21**(8):3447-3453. DOI: 10.1200/JCO.2003.01.096

[81] Clifford GM, Polesel J, Rickenbach M, et al. For the Swiss HIV Cohort. Cancer risk in the Swiss HIV cohort study: Associations with immunodeficiency, smoking, and highly active antiretroviral therapy. Journal of the National Cancer Institute. 2005;**97**(6):425-432. DOI: 10.1093/jnci/dji072

[82] Stein H, Hummel M. Hodgkin's disease: Biology and origins of Hodgkin and reed-Sternberg cells. Cancer Treatment Reviews. 1999;**25**(3):161-168. DOI: 10.1053/ctrv.1999.0117

[83] Chan WC. The reed-Sternberg cells in classical Hodgkin's disease. Hematological Oncology. 2001;**19**(1): 1-17. DOI: 10.1002/hon.659

[84] Leigton RA, Pivnik AV, Sergeeva EP, et al. Plasma cell neoplasms in HIV-Infected patients: A literature review and case series. Clinical Oncohematology. 2017;**10**(4):464-470. DOI: 10.21320/2500-2139-2017-10-4-464-470